Life, Death and the Immune System

. . .

SCIENTIFIC AMERICAN: A SPECIAL ISSUE

W. H. FREEMAN AND COMPANY
New York

Library of Congress Cataloging-in-Publication Data

Life, death and the immune system : Scientific American:
   A special issue.
         p.   cm.
      "Originally appeared as articles and the closing
   essay in the September 1993 issue of Scientific
   American."
      Includes bibliographical references and index.
      ISBN 0-7167-2547-9
      1. Immune system.   2. Immunity   3. Immunologic
   diseases.
   I. Scientific American.
   QR181.L53   1994
   616.07'9—dc20   93-37556
                                                         CIP

Printed in the United States of America

1 2 3 4 5 6 7 8 9 0 RRD 9 9 8 7 6 5 4 3

CONTENTS

FOREWORD

Ask someone what aspect of his or her being is most essential to that person's unique identity and the reply is likely to be: my mind, or my consciousness. Perhaps, but the immune system might turn out to be a stronger candidate. From before birth until death the system, like the porter who excludes nonmembers from a exclusive club, continuously draws distinctions between entities that are part of an individual's physiology and those that are not. This republication of the September 1993 issue of *Scientific American* provides an authoritative portrait of this most dynamic and powerful field of medical and biological research.

Through cells called *B* lymphocytes the system has the ability to recognize millions of kinds of alien proteins. When it encounters one, perhaps in the form of the coat of a virus or the glycoprotein-studded surface of a bacterium's cell membrane, it unleashes what is usually a devastating attack. The primary agents of destruction are *T* lymphocytes, granulocytes and neutrophils. Aided by complement and other defensive compounds in the blood, these cells engulf and digest invaders or destroy them by releasing a barrage of toxic compounds.

Yet the system spares the host's own tissues this biochemical savagery. During the months before birth, the developing immune system learns to recognize and avoid attacking the body's own tissues, which bear characteristic major histocompatibility complex (MHC) molecules. MHC molecules are the body's own monogram. Unless an individual belongs to a pair of identical twins, the chance of anyone else sporting the same cluster of MHC molecules is literally astronomical. Immune system cells that would participate in an attack on tissue bearing the host's MHC molecules are eliminated or rendered inactive.

No system is perfect, not even the marvelously complex immune system. The controls that prevent *T* cells, macrophages and other cellular agents of immunity from attacking host tissue can fail. Or an antigen can so closely resemble host tissue that the attacking cells do not distinguish friend from foe—a biological analogue to "friendly fire." Such malfunction precipitates multiple sclerosis, rheumatoid arthritis, systemic lupus, myasthenia gravis and a depressingly long list of other autoimmune diseases.

Sometimes the immune system can act too zealously. Defense against parasites depends on the ability to produce large amounts of an antibody, immunoglobulin E (IgE). In the artificial environment of industrial society, parasites seldom threaten anyone's health. Bereft of its primary target, IgE, produced in copious amounts, triggers allergic reactions to other, relatively benign antigens lurking in the external environment or diet.

In immunology as in other disciplines, knowledge is power. Exquisite understanding of the immune system's structure and function has enabled researchers to begin to equip clinicians with powerful weapons against autoimmune disease, infectious disease and allergy. New weapons against cancer and deft ways to induce the acceptance of surgical grafts are in prospect. The immune system itself, clinicians are discovering, is a powerful medical and surgical implement.

Disease, however, has not yet forfeited the last laugh. AIDS so far resists all efforts at chemical treatment or prevention. Still some comfort can be taken. Had HIV struck even 10 years earlier not enough would have been known about the immune system to begin to understand what was happening to the disease's victims. Now we at least know where and how to look for a way to control this ultimate pathogen.

What are our prospects for survival? Presuming that our species can weather AIDS, will the immune system retain the upper hand against other diseases, as it has done for at least the past 200,000 years? By itself, that record provides grounds for optimism. The game between human and microbe, however, is open-ended. Bacteria and viruses, like their hosts, continue to evolve. In addition to HIV, several other new pathogens have emerged in the last fifteen or so years. The human population continues to grow dramatically, bringing more people into contact with one another than ever before. Jet aircraft and other forms of high-speed transportation enable man (or woman) and microbe to move easily from one distant part of the world to another.

Although the immune system will probably not elaborate itself in any dramatically novel way, its unspent reserves of recognition and resistance provide reason to be optimistic. So does vigorous, global basic research into the structure and function of immunity. If we as a species can organize our social and economic order to deliver the benefits of the work of immunologists to everyone who needs them, we have sound reason to hope for a viable future.

Jonathan Piel
For the Board of Editors

Life, Death and the Immune System

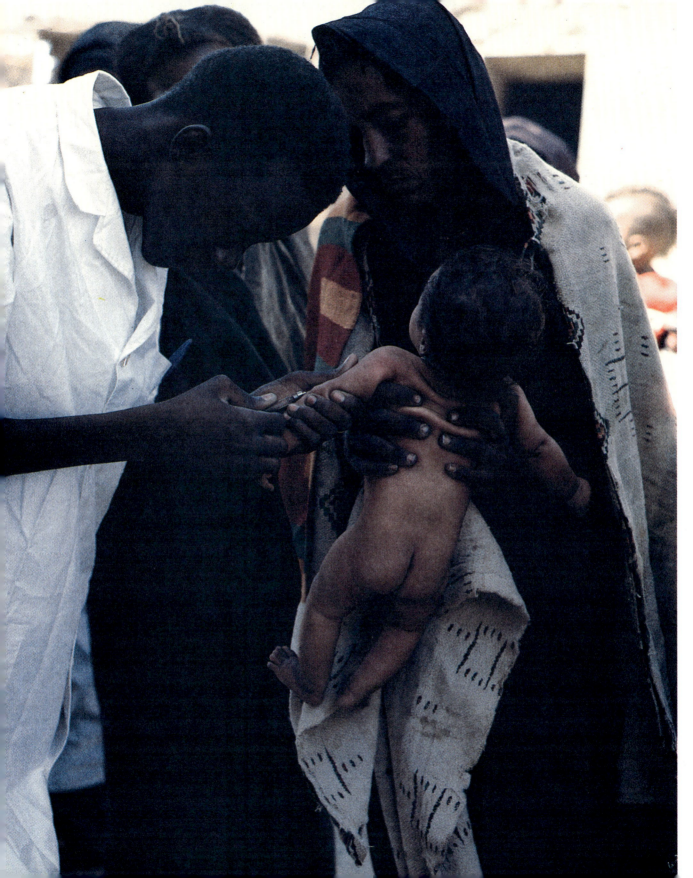

Life, Death and the Immune System

By defining and defending the self, the immune system makes life possible; malfunction causes illness and death. Study of the system provides a unifying view of biology.

. . .

Sir Gustav J. V. Nossal

What did Franz Schubert, John Keats and Elizabeth Barrett Browning have in common? Each was a creative genius, but each also had his or her life tragically shortened by a communicable disease that today could have been prevented or cured. Progress in the treatment of such diseases undoubtedly ranks as one of the greatest achievements of modern science. Smallpox has been completely eradicated, and poliomyelitis and measles may be problems of the past by the end of the century. So great has been the headway against infectious diseases that until the current AIDS pandemic, industrialized countries had placed them on the back burner among major national concerns (see Figure 1.1).

Such staggering improvements in public health alone would justify tremendous efforts to understand the human immune system. Yet the field of immunology embraces more than just the nature and prevention of infections. Immunologic research is pointing toward new approaches for treating cancer and diseases that result from

Figure 1.1 WIDESPREAD VACCINATION of infants in Nigeria and in other developing countries has drastically reduced the incidence of diseases such as diphtheria and poliomyelitis. That worldwide assault on infectious disease has been one of the triumphs of modern immunology.

lapses or malfunctions in the immune response. This work also provides a scientific framework for examining the chemical organization of living systems and integrating that information into an understanding of how the organism functions as a whole.

I am a little ashamed to admit that I did not immediately recognize the underlying importance of immunology. As a medical student in the 1950s, I became interested in viruses, hoping that the analysis of their growth might reveal the most profound details of the life process. I aspired to study under Sir Frank Macfarlane Burnet, the prominent Australian virologist, at the Walter and Eliza Hall Institute of Medical Research in Melbourne.

After my graduation and hospital training, I was lucky enough to be accepted. Burnet wrote, however, that he had become interested less in viruses than in exploring the human immune system. I was utterly dismayed. To my thinking, the early giants—Louis Pasteur, Paul Ehrlich and Emil A. von Behring—had already discovered the fundamental truths about immunity (see Figure 1.2). Public health, the major application of immunology research, seemed the dullest of the subjects in the medical curriculum.

Since then I have learned how wrong I was. Just as I began my graduate work, a series of immune-related discoveries began ushering in an

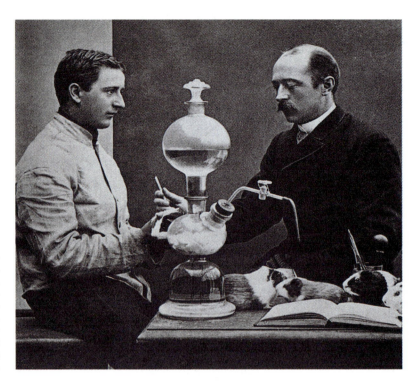

Figure 1.2 EMIL A. VON BEHRING (*right*) **studied the effects of antitoxins that appear in the bloodstream after an infection; he coined the term "antibody" to describe them. Von Behring's experiments on inducing immunity in laboratory animals led to the development of an antibody serum to prevent diphtheria. In 1901 he received the first Nobel Prize in medicine for that work.**

extraordinary chapter in the history of biomedicine. Researchers observed that the white blood cells called lymphocytes, which destroy pathogenic microbes that enter the body, can attack cancer cells and hold them in check, at least temporarily. Other experiments showed that those same lymphocytes can also behave in less desirable ways. For example, they can act against the foreign cells in transplanted organs and cause graft rejection. If the regulation of the immune system breaks down, lymphocytes can attack cells belonging to the very body that they should be protecting, leading to a potentially fatal autoimmune disease.

All these findings intensified interest in one of the most central and baffling mysteries of the immune system: how it is able to recognize the seemingly infinite number of viruses, bacteria and other foreign elements that threaten the health of the organism. In most biochemical interactions, such as the binding of a hormone to a receptor or the adhesion of a virus to its host cell, eons of evolution have refined the chemistry involved so that each molecule unites with its partner in a precise, predetermined way. The immune system, in contrast, cannot anticipate what foreign molecule it will confront next.

One of the crucial elements that helps the immune system meet that challenge is antibody, a large protein molecule discovered in 1890 by von Behring and Shibasaburo Kitasato. Antibodies latch onto and neutralize foreign invaders such as bacteria and viruses; they also coat microbes in a way that makes them palatable to scavenger cells, such as macrophages. Each type of antibody acts on only a very specific target molecule, known as an antigen (see boxed figure "How the Immune System Defends the Body"). Consequently, antibodies that attack anthrax bacilli have no effect against typhoid. For decades, biologists thought of the antigen as a kind of template around which the antibody molecule molded itself to assume a complementary form. This theory, first clearly articulated by Felix Haurowitz in the 1930s and later espoused by Linus Pauling, held sway until about 1960.

By the mid-1960s the template model was in trouble. Gordon L. Ada of the Hall Institute and I

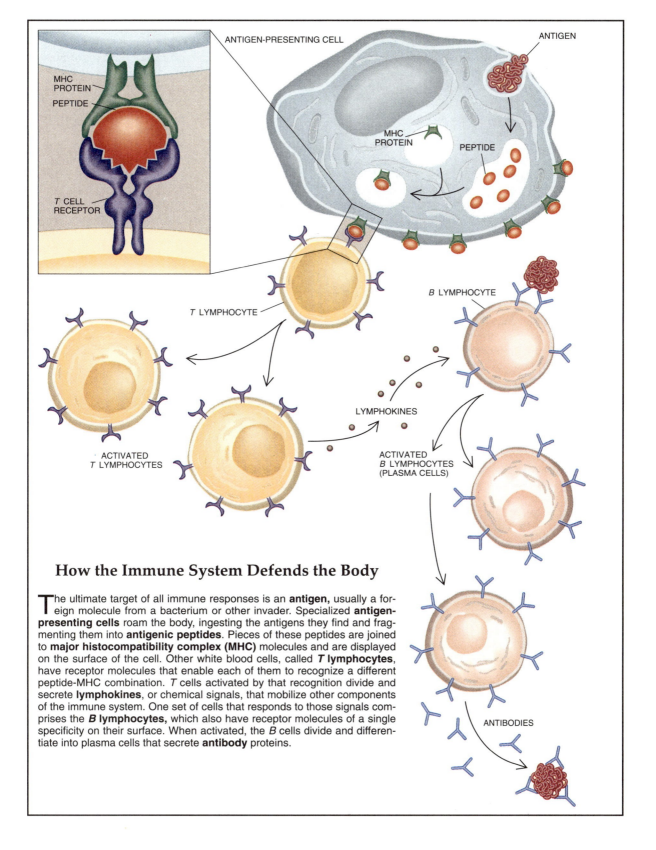

ANTIGEN-PRESENTING CELL

ANTIGEN

MHC PROTEIN

PEPTIDE

T CELL RECEPTOR

MHC PROTEIN

PEPTIDE

T LYMPHOCYTE

B LYMPHOCYTE

ACTIVATED T LYMPHOCYTES

LYMPHOKINES

ACTIVATED B LYMPHOCYTES (PLASMA CELLS)

ANTIBODIES

How the Immune System Defends the Body

The ultimate target of all immune responses is an **antigen,** usually a foreign molecule from a bacterium or other invader. Specialized **antigen-presenting cells** roam the body, ingesting the antigens they find and fragmenting them into **antigenic peptides**. Pieces of these peptides are joined to **major histocompatibility complex (MHC)** molecules and are displayed on the surface of the cell. Other white blood cells, called **T lymphocytes**, have receptor molecules that enable each of them to recognize a different peptide-MHC combination. T cells activated by that recognition divide and secrete **lymphokines**, or chemical signals, that mobilize other components of the immune system. One set of cells that responds to those signals comprises the **B lymphocytes,** which also have receptor molecules of a single specificity on their surface. When activated, the B cells divide and differentiate into plasma cells that secrete **antibody** proteins.

demonstrated that antibody-making cells did not contain any antigen around which to shape an antibody. Studies of enzymes showed that the structure of a protein depends only on the particular sequence of its amino acid subunits. Furthermore, Francis Crick deduced that, in biological systems, information flows from DNA to RNA to protein. For this reason, antigen proteins could not define new antibody proteins: the information for the antibody structures had to be encoded in the genes. Those findings raised a puzzling question: If genes dictate the manufacture of antibodies, how can there be specific genes for each of the millions of different antibodies that the body can fabricate?

In 1955 Niels K. Jerne, then at the California Institute of Technology, had already hit on a possible explanation for the incredible diversity of antibodies. He suggested that the immune response is selective rather than instructive—that is, mammals have an inherent capacity to synthesize billions of different antibodies and that the arrival of an antigen only accelerates the formation of the antibody that makes the best fit.

Two years later Burnet and David W. Talmage of the University of Colorado independently hypothesized that antibodies sit on the surface of lymphocytes and that each lymphocyte bears only one kind of antibody. When a foreign antigen enters the body, it eventually encounters a lymphocyte having a matching receptor and chemically stimulates it to divide and to mass-produce the relevant antibody. In 1958 Joshua Lederberg, then visiting the Hall Institute, and I demonstrated that when an animal is immunized with two different antigens, any given cell does in fact make just one type of antibody.

Soon thereafter Gerald M. Edelman of the Rockefeller University and Rodney R. Porter of the University of Oxford discovered that antibodies are composed of four small proteins called chains. Each antibody possesses two identical heavy chains and two identical light chains. An intertwining light chain and heavy chain form an active site capable of recognizing an antigen, so each antibody molecule has two identical recognition sites. Knowing that two chains contribute to the binding site helps to explain the great diversity of antibodies because of the large number of possible pair combinations.

A set of experiments initiated by Susumu Tonegawa of the Basel Institute for Immunology led to the definitive description of how the immune system can produce so many different antibody types. He found that, unlike nearly all other genes in the body, those that contain the code for the heavy chains do not preexist in the fertilized egg. Instead the code resides in four sets of mini-genes located in widely separated parts of the nucleus. Antibody diversity springs from the size of these mini-gene families: there are more than 100 kinds of V (variable) genes, 12 D (diversity) genes and four J (joining) genes. The C, or constant, genes vary in ways that affect only the function of the antibody, not its antigen affinity.

During the development of an antibody-forming cell, one member from each set of mini-genes jumps out of its original position and links with the other jumpers to form a complete V-D-J-C gene. This genetic rearrangement allows for 4,800 different varieties ($100 \times 12 \times 4 \times 1$) of heavy chains. The same process occurs in the assembly of the light-chain genes, except that they have only V, J and C segments, so there are about 400 basic combinations for them. The diversity of heavy and light chains allows for the existence of $4,800 \times 400$, or 1,920,000, antibody genes. Moreover, special enzymes can insert a few extra DNA coding units at the junctions between the V and D or D and J segments when they interlink, which further increases the number of possible antibody constructions.

Despite their enormous versatility, antibodies alone cannot provide full protection from infectious attack. Some diseases, such as tuberculosis, slip inside their host cells so quickly that they can hide from antibody molecules. In these cases, a second form of immune response comes into play. When the infected cells become inflamed, lymphocytes attack them so as to confine the infection. This defense mechanism is known as cell-mediated immunity, in contrast with the so-called humoral immunity mediated by antibodies.

In the early 1960s Jacques F.A.P. Miller, then at the Chester Beatty Research Institute in London, and Noel L. Warner and Aleksander Szenberg of the Hall Institute determined that lymphocytes fall into two different classes, each of which controls one of the two types of immune response. Cell-mediated immunity involves a type of lymphocyte that originates in the thymus and is thus called a *T* cell. Humoral immunity occurs through the action of antibodies, which are produced by the lymphocytes known as B cells that form in the bone marrow (see boxed figure "The Decentralized Defenses of Immunity").

T cells and B cells differ not only in their function but also in the way they locate a foreign invader. As Talmage and Burnet hypothesized, B cells can recognize antigens because they carry antibodies on their surface. Each T cell also has a unique receptor, but unlike B cells, T cells cannot "see" the entire antigen. Instead the receptors on T cells recognize protein fragments of antigens, or peptides, linear sequences of eight to 15 amino acids. T cells spot foreign peptide sequences on the surface of body cells, including bits of virus, mutated molecules in cancer cells or even sections of the inner part of a microbe. A molecule known as a major histocompatibility complex (MHC) protein brings the peptide to the cell surface, where the T cell can bind to it.

T cells and antibodies make perfect partners (see Figure 1.3). Antibodies respond swiftly to toxin molecules and to the outer surfaces of microbes; T cells discover the antigens of hidden inner pathogens, which makes them particularly effective at tracking down infectious agents. For instance, a virus might be able, through mutation, to change its outer envelope rapidly and in this way frustrate neutralization by antibodies. That same virus might contain within its core several proteins that are so essential to its life process that mutations are not permitted. When that virus replicates inside cells, short peptide chains from those viral proteins break off and travel to the cell surface. They serve as ripe targets for the T cell, which can then attack the infected cell and inhibit the spread of the virus.

So far I have described T and B lymphocytes as though they operate independently, but in actuality they form a tightly interwoven system. T cells make close contact with B cells, stimulate them into an active state and secrete lymphokines, molecules that promote antibody formation. T cells also can suppress antibody formation by releasing inhibitory lymphokines.

B cells, in turn, process antigens into the form to which T cells most readily respond, attach the antigens to MHC molecules and display them on the cell surface (see Figure 1.4). In this way, B cells help to stimulate T cells into an active state. Researchers have observed that B cells can also inhibit T cell responses under experimental conditions. Such highly regulated positive and negative

feedback loops are a hallmark of the organization of the immune system.

The specialization of the immune system does not end with its division into B and T cells. T cells themselves comprise two subpopulations, CD4 (helper) and CD8 (killer) T cells. CD4 cells recognize peptides from proteins that have been taken up by macrophages and other specialized antigen-capturing cells. CD8 cells react to samples of peptides originating within a cell itself, such as a segment of a virus in an infected cell or mutant proteins in a cancer cell. Each variety of T cell utilizes its own form of MHC to make the peptides noticeable.

When CD4 T cells encounter the proper chemical signal, they produce large amounts of lymphokines to accelerate the division of other T cells and to promote inflammation. Some CD4 cells specialize in helping B cells, others in causing inflammation. Activated CD8 cells produce much smaller amounts of lymphokines but develop the capacity to punch holes into target cells and to secrete chemicals that kill infected cells, limiting the spread of a virus. Because of their murderous nature, CD8 T cells are also referred to as cytotoxic T cells.

B cells undergo an especially stunning transformation once activated (see Figure 1.5). Before it meets antigen, the B cell is a small cell having a compact nucleus and very little cytoplasm—a head office without much happening on the factory floor. When the cell springs into action, it divides repeatedly and builds up thousands of assembly points in its cytoplasm for the manufacture of antibodies, as well as an extensive channeling system for packaging and exporting the antibodies. One B cell can pump out more than 10 million antibody molecules an hour.

My co-workers and I routinely cultivate a single B cell to grow a "clone" comprising hundreds of daughter cells. After one week, those clones can generate 100 billion identical antibody molecules to study. Such clonal cultures have enabled us to witness another of the B cell's remarkable talents. B cells can switch from making one isotype, or functional variety, of antibody to another without changing the antigen to which the antibody binds. Each isotype of an antibody derives from a different form of the C mini-gene.

Each antibody isotype has its own peculiar advantage. One isotype serves as a first line of defense; another specializes in neutralizing toxins; a

The Decentralized Defenses of Immunity

Lymphocytes, which are responsible for specific immunity, are born in the **primary lymphoid organs:** the **thymus** makes *T* cells, and the **bone marrow** makes *B* cells. The cells circulate in the blood until they reach one of the numerous **secondary lymphoid organs,** such as the **lymph nodes, spleen** and **tonsils**. They then exit the bloodstream through specialized blood vessels called **high endothelial venules**. The nodes are excellent places for lymphocytes to become activated by antigens and antigen-presenting cells entering through the **afferent lymphatic vessels**. *T* cells generally become activated by antigen in the **paracortex;** activated *B* cells become antibody-producing plasma cells in areas such as the **germinal centers of the lymphoid follicles**. Activated lymphocytes flow out of the nodes through the **efferent lymphatics** and travel to the bloodstream.

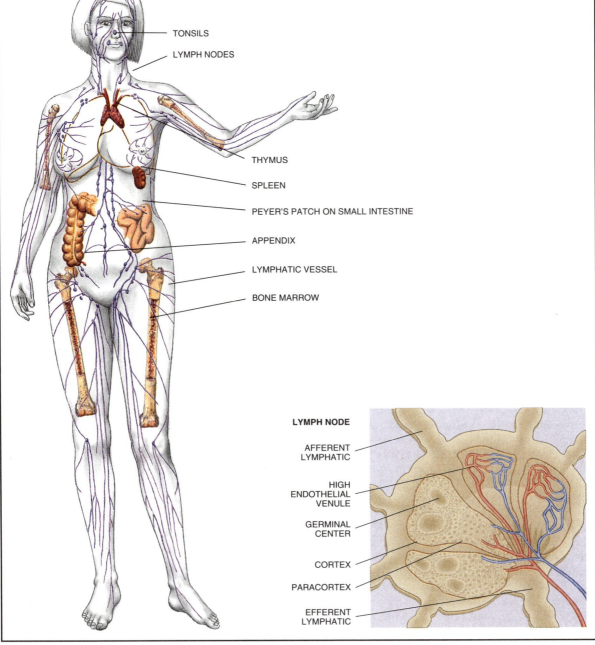

TONSILS

LYMPH NODES

THYMUS

SPLEEN

PEYER'S PATCH ON SMALL INTESTINE

APPENDIX

LYMPHATIC VESSEL

BONE MARROW

LYMPH NODE

AFFERENT LYMPHATIC

HIGH ENDOTHELIAL VENULE

GERMINAL CENTER

CORTEX

PARACORTEX

EFFERENT LYMPHATIC

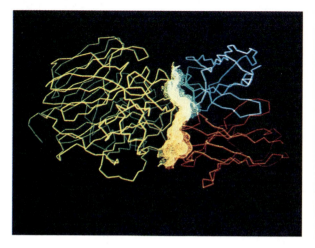
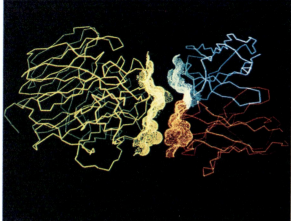

Figure 1.3 ANTIGEN AND ANTIBODY fit together tightly, like two hands shaking (*left*). This computer simulation, based on x-ray crystallography data collected by Peter M. Colman and William R. Tulip of CSIRO in Melbourne, shows an antigen from an influenza virus (*left side*) interacting with an antibody (*right side*), as happens on the surface of a *B* lymphocyte. Separating the two molecules by a distance of eight angstroms reveals their complementary surfaces (*right*). The variable part of the heavy protein chain is shown as red, the corresponding part of the light chain as blue.

third suffuses mucus and so helps to create a barrier against infectious agents attempting to enter through the nose, throat or intestines. In response to lymphokines from *T* cells, *B* cells can switch from one isotype of antibody to another within a day or so.

Both *B* and *T* lymphocytes get a helping hand from various other cells and molecules. When antibodies attach to a bacterium, they can activate complement, a class of enzymes that kill bacteria by destroying their outer membranes. Some lymphokines send out a chemical call to macrophages, granulocytes and other white blood cells that clean up the mess at an infected site by gobbling up germs and dead cells. Such tidiness is enormously important: a patient having no granulocytes faces grave risk of death from the infectious bacteria that feed on cellular corpses. Clearly, all the white blood cells work together as a well-orchestrated team.

Amid all the complex operations of the immune defenses, it is utterly crucial that lymphocytes remain consistently benign toward the body's own cells, commonly referred to as self, while reacting aggressively to those that it recognizes as foreign, or nonself. Burnet postulated that self-recognition is not genetically determined but rather is learned by the immune system during the organism's embryonic stage. He suggested that a foreign antigen introduced into an embryo before the immune system had developed would trick the lymphocytes into regarding the foreign molecule as self. Burnet's attempts to prove his theory by injecting an influenza vaccine into chick embryos did not elicit the expected null response, however.

In 1953 Rupert E. Billingham, Leslie Brent and Sir Peter B. Medawar, working at University College, London, succeeded where Burnet had failed. The three men were exploring ways to transplant skin from one individual to another—in order, for instance, to treat a burn victim. Medawar had previously discovered that the body rejected such skin grafts because of an immune response. When he came across Burnet's theoretical writings, Medawar and his colleagues set about injecting inbred mouse embryos with spleen-derived cells from a different mouse strain. Some embryos died as a result of this insult, but those that survived to adulthood accepted skin grafts from the donor strain. A patch of black fur growing on a white mouse dramatically showcased the discovery of actively acquired immunologic tolerance; for the first time, lymphocytes were fooled into recognizing nonself as self. Burnet and Medawar shared a Nobel Prize for their work.

Subsequent research clarified why Burnet's experiment had gone awry. Medawar's group used

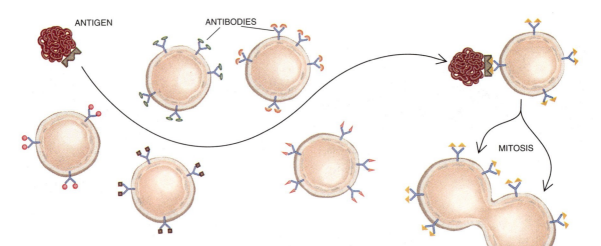

ANTIGEN

ANTIBODIES

MITOSIS

ACTIVATED *B* LYMPHOCYTE

ANTIBODIES

Figure 1.4 CLONAL SELECTION enables the immune system to react to a myriad of possible pathogens. Lymphocytes having any one of millions of different surface antibodies constantly roam the body. When the antigen on the surface of a foreign entity meets a lymphocyte having a matching antibody (*top*), the lymphocyte swells and begins to divide rapidly (*right*). Once they reach maturity, *B* cells secrete antibodies that attack the invader (*bottom*); *T* cells generate lymphokines, chemicals that boost the activity of other cells in the immune system.

living cells as an antigen source—specifically, cells that could move into critical locations such as the thymus and the bone marrow. As long as those donor cells lived, they continued to make antigens that influenced the emerging lymphocytes. Burnet's influenza vaccine, on the other hand, had been rapidly consumed and broken down by scavenger cells; not enough antigen reached the immune system to induce a significant degree of tolerance.

The realization that immune response depends heavily on the vast diversity of antibodies on the body's innumerable *B* cells suggested the mechanism by which lymphocytes learn to ignore cells of the self. An immune reaction represents the activation of specific lymphocytes selected from the body's varied repertoire. It seemed logical that tolerance of self could be seen as the mirror image of immunity: the systematic deletion of those cells that respond to self-antigen.

Genetic influences and environmental triggers can cause the usual immunologic rules to break down. In those instances, *B* cells or *T* cells, or both, may respond to self-antigens, attacking the body's own cells and leading to a devastating autoimmune disease. Some such disorders result from misdirected antibodies: in hemolytic anemia, antibodies attack red blood cells, and in myasthenia

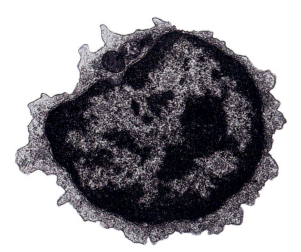

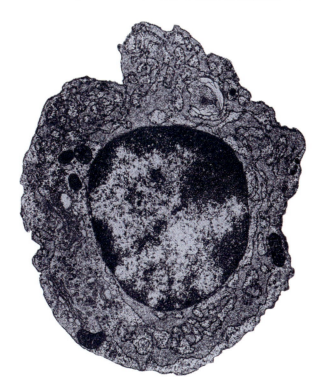

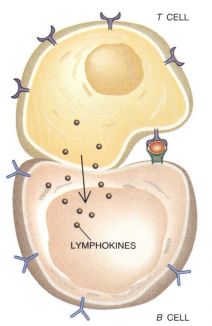

T CELL

LYMPHOKINES

B CELL

Figure 1.5 *B* LYMPHOCYTE in its resting state is little more than a nucleus surrounded by a thin enclosure of cytoplasm (*top left*). Once a *B* cell meets a matching antigen, it develops an extended body (*top right*) containing polyribosomes, which make antibodies, and an elaborate channel system for exporting those antibodies. *T* lymphocytes can regu⌐ 'e the behavior of *B* cells by administering lymphokines through an intimate junction somewhat like a nerve synapse (*bottom*). During these interactions, the *B* cell can also influence the activity of the *T* cell.

gravis, antibodies turn on a vital protein on muscle cells that receives signals from nerves. *T* cells play the villain's role in other autoimmune diseases: in insulin-dependent diabetes, *T* lymphocytes destroy insulin-producing cells in the pancreas, and in multiple sclerosis, they direct their fury against the insulation surrounding nerve fibers in the brain and spinal cord.

Treating autoimmune diseases necessitates abolishing or at least restraining the immune system.

Immunosuppressive and anti-inflammatory drugs can achieve the desired effect, but such a blunderbuss approach suppresses not only the bad, antiself response but also all the desirable immune reactions. Fortunately, researchers are making some progress toward the ideal goal of reestablishing specific immunologic tolerance to the beleaguered self-antigen.

One kind of therapy involves feeding the patient large quantities of the attacked self-antigen;

surprisingly enough, such an approach can selectively restrain future responses to that antigen. Researchers have achieved similar results by administering antigens intravenously while the T cells are temporarily blindfolded by monoclonal antibodies that block their antigen receptors. Some treatments for autoimmune diseases based on these approaches have reached the stage of clinical trials.

Successful organ transplantation also requires shutting down an undesired aspect of immune response. In principle, the surgeon can begin supplying immunosuppressive drugs at the time of surgery, preempting a lymphocyte attack. Most organ transplants provoke such a strong T cell response that the doses of drugs needed to prevent organ rejection are even higher than those used to treat autoimmune diseases. Fortunately, those dosages can be reduced after a few months. Newer, more powerful immunosuppressive drugs are leading to good success rates for transplants of the kidney, heart, liver, bone marrow, heart-lung and pancreas; recently a few small-bowel transplants have taken. Researchers are also striving to develop targeted drugs that dampen the organ rejection response while still allowing the body to react to infectious diseases.

Transplantation has become so successful that doctors often confront a shortage of organs from recently deceased donors. Workers therefore are renewing their efforts to perform xenotransplantation, the transplantation of organs from animal donors. Tissue from endocrine glands can be cultured so that it loses some of its antigenic punch, raising the possibility that insulin-secreting cells from pigs will one day be grafted into diabetics. Chemical treatments may be able to "humanize" crucial molecules in animal organs so as to ameliorate the ferocity of immune rejection. Nevertheless, xenotransplantation faces formidable technical and ethical obstacles.

Immunologic attacks on tissues in the body need not be horrific; they could actually be beneficial if directed against cancers. Indeed, one controversial theory—the immune surveillance theory, first articulated by Lewis Thomas when he was at New York University—holds that eliminating precancerous cells is one of the prime duties of the constantly patrolling lymphocytes.

People whose immune system has been suppressed by drugs—mostly recipients of organ transplants—do in fact experience a higher incidence of leukemias, lymphomas and skin cancers fairly soon after transplantation than do similar individuals in the general population. After three decades of observing kidney transplant patients, physicians find that those individuals also experience a somewhat elevated susceptibility to many common cancers, such as those of the lung, breast, colon, uterus and prostate. These findings hint that immune surveillance may act to hold at least certain cancers in check. Alternatively, drug-associated cancers may be the result of some mechanism other than immunosuppression.

Further evidence of the immune system's role in preventing cancer comes from studies of mouse cancers induced by viruses or by chemical carcinogens. Those cancers often provoke strong immune responses when transplanted into genetically identical mice, which proves that the cancerous cells bear antigens that mark them as abnormal. Spontaneously arising cancers in mice, which are likely to be more akin to human cancer, provoke little or no immune response, however.

Yet even spontaneous cancers may carry some tumor-specific antigens that could arouse a reaction from the immune system if other chemical signals are present. One highly potent trigger molecule is known as B7. When inserted into the cells of a tumor, B7 can convert deadly, uncontrollable cancer cells into ones that T cells attack and destroy. B7 is not itself an antigen, but it evidently helps antigenic molecules in the tumor cell to activate T cells (see Figure 1.6).

The discovery of immunostimulating molecules such as B7 has renewed interest in the possibility of developing anticancer vaccines. Such treatments might be effective against malignant melanoma, the cancer arising from pigmented moles. These cancers contain a family of proteins collectively called MAGE, which has been extensively studied by Thierry Boon at the Ludwig Institute for Cancer Research in Brussels. In laboratory experiments, a peptide derived from MAGE can provoke a strong attack from cytotoxic T cells. If researchers could learn how to manipulate the antigen properly—perhaps by injecting a patient with MAGE or its constituent peptides, along with molecules designed to strengthen immunity—they might be able to create an effective therapy for melanoma.

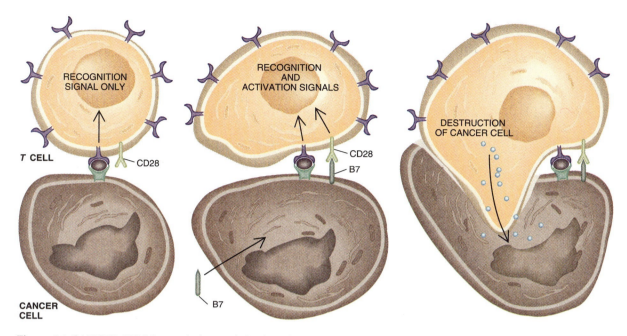

Figure 1.6 CANCER CELLS can elude attack by lymphocytes even if they bear distinctive antigens. That absence of immune response may occur because cancerous cells lack the proper costimulatory molecules (*left*). Researchers are attempting to induce the body to fight tumors by inserting the molecule B7 into cancer cells (*center*). When B7 engages CD28, a complementary molecule on the surface of *T* cells, it generates a signal that instigates an assault on the cancer cells (*right*).

Another way to fight cancers involves boosting the immune response to aberrant forms of a class of proteins known as mucins. Normal mucins consist of a protein core almost completely enveloped by a shell of sugar molecules. Many cancerous cells, most notably those associated with tumors of the gastrointestinal tract, lung or ovary, contain altered mucins whose cores are exposed. Workers have identified peptides from the core proteins in mucins to which *T* cells strongly respond. Vaccines constructed from those peptides may be able to induce cytotoxic *T* cells to attack the naked core proteins and thereby kill the cancerous cells.

Devising cancer vaccines presents a difficult challenge. Tumor cells have a great capacity to mutate, which allows them to avoid destruction by discarding or changing their distinctive antigens. Killing every single tumor cell, as must be done to cure cancer, will not be easy in advanced cases of cancer. And yet experimental vaccines have shown tantalizing signs of success. In tests on patients who had several forms of widespread cancer, such as melanoma, kidney cancer and certain forms of leukemia, roughly one fifth of them experienced a dramatic regression of their tumors in response to these vaccines. Little is known about why those people responded and others did not.

Many workers believe cancer vaccines will come into their own as weapons against the few mutant cells that persist in the body after cancer surgery, chemotherapy or radiation therapy. These surviving cells can cause a recurrence of the cancer even after an apparently successful primary therapy. In principle, killing the few million cancer cells that remain after a primary treatment should be easier than eliminating the hundreds of billions that exist beforehand.

Despite the promise of such innovative techniques, new and improved vaccines against infectious disease continue to be the most urgent and immediate application of immunologic research. In this arena, the World Health Organization's Expanded Program on Immunization (EPI) has stood out as a laudable triumph amid the generally troubled global public health scene. With wonderful help from UNICEF, the World Bank, Rotary International and the developing countries' health authorities, EPI provides protection against six major diseases—diphtheria, whooping cough, tetanus, poliomyelitis, measles and tuberculosis—to over 80 percent of the more than 100 million children born every year in the Third World.

Last year EPI added hepatitis B vaccine to its list, although cost considerations have limited the number of doses available. In many Asian and African countries, 5 to 10 percent of the population become chronic carriers of the hepatitis B virus; a significant proportion of these acquire severe liver disease and finally liver cancer. An infant who receives the vaccine at birth does not become a carrier and is protected from the virus. Mass vaccination against hepatitis B is worthwhile even in Western countries, not only because of the risk faced by homosexual men but also because many of these countries now include significant Asian or African-derived populations.

Encouraging though the trends are, an enormous amount remains to be done in the realm of immunization. Effective vaccines against several forms of meningitis are not yet in widespread use. The available vaccines against typhoid, cholera, tuberculosis and influenza are only partially effective. No generally available vaccine exists for many common diseases, such as pneumonia, diarrhea, malaria and cancers caused by human papillomavirus and glandular fever virus. Furthermore, rich and poor countries alike face the practical problems of delivering the vaccine to those who need it and making sure that it is used. The World Health Organization badly needs extra funds to sustain its marvelous thrust in research and deployment.

Devising a vaccine against AIDS is one of the most urgent and daunting tasks facing immunology researchers. There are now at least 10 million people around the world infected with the human immunodeficiency virus (HIV), which causes AIDS; most of these people live in developing countries. HIV manifests a dizzying capacity to mutate, and it can hide from the immune system inside lymphocytes and scavenger cells. Still, there are some encouraging signs that the virus can be defeated. HIV often lies dormant in humans for years, which suggests that immune processes hold the virus in check for long periods. Antibodies can neutralize HIV, and cytotoxic T cells can kill at least some of the virus-carrying cells. Vaccines have prevented AIDS-like infections in monkeys. It will take several years, however, to determine whether any of the present clinical trials hold real promise.

The AIDS crisis has so enhanced public awareness of immunology that when I attend social or business functions and reveal that I am an immunologist, people commonly respond, "Oh, then you must be working on AIDS!" They are often surprised to hear that immunology is a vast science that predates the identification of AIDS by many decades.

And yet the interdisciplinary nature of immunology has had, I believe, a significant salutary effect on all the biological sciences. When I was young, many researchers worried that as the specialties and subspecialties bloomed, scientists would discover more and more about less and less, so that the research enterprise would splinter into myriad fragments, each bright and shiny in its own right but having little connection to the others.

Rather a new, integrated biology has arisen, built on the foundation of molecular biology, protein chemistry and cell biology, encompassing fields as diverse as neurobiology, developmental biology, endocrinology, cancer research and cardiovascular physiology. A fundamental finding made within one discipline spreads like wildfire through the others.

Immunology sits at the center of the action. The cells of the immune system constitute ideal tools for basic biological research. They grow readily in the test tube, display a rich diversity of chemical receptors and manufacture molecules of great specificity and power; consequently, the lymphocyte is perhaps the best understood of all living cells. Moreover, immunology embraces many interlinked molecular and cellular systems and considers how they affect the organism as a whole. As a result, the immune system has become an instructive model of the life process. Enough of the master plan has been revealed to provide a sturdy springboard for future research, but enough remains hidden to challenge the most intrepid explorer.

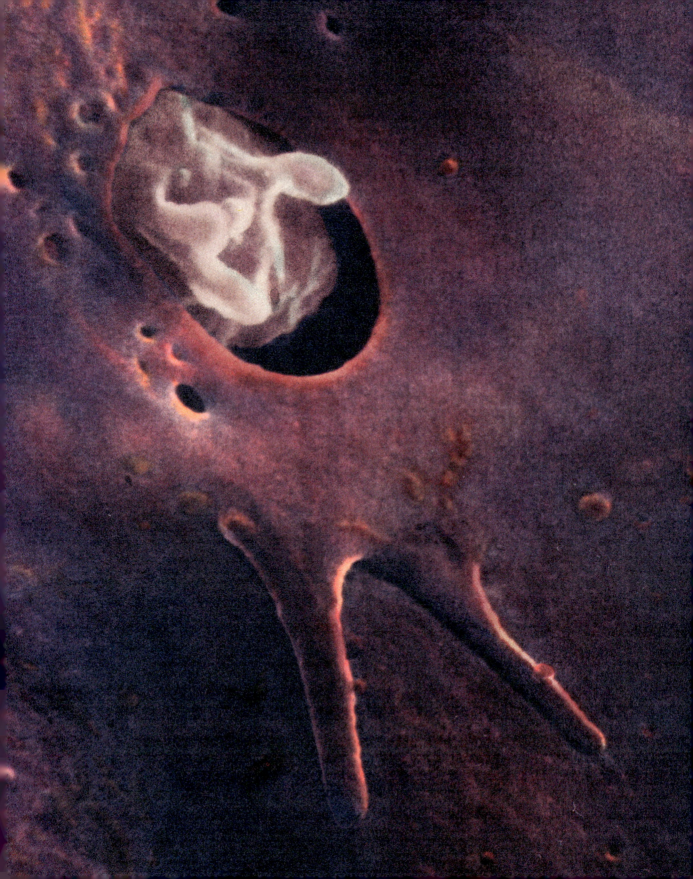

How the Immune System Develops

Environmental and genetic signals cue cells as they differentiate into the many lineages that recognize foreign antigens and fight off invaders.

. . .

Irving L. Weissman and Max D. Cooper

The marvelous array of deftly interacting cells that defend the body against microbial and viral invaders arises from a few precursor cells that first appear about nine weeks after conception. From that point onward, the cells of the immune system go through a continuously repeated cycle of development. The stem cells on which the immune system depends both reproduce themselves and give rise to many specialized lineages— B cells, macrophages, killer T cells, helper T cells, inflammatory T cells and others.

The cells of the immune system are not isolated in a single space or arrayed in the form of a single organ; instead they exist as potentially mobile entities, unattached to other cells. This characteristic is not only crucial to their function but also confers a boon on researchers, who can isolate immune cells in relatively pure form at every stage of differentiation. Experimenters can thus determine the properties of cells and construct cellular "family trees," or lineages.

The information gained in this way serves biologists attempting to understand the general subject of how cells develop and differentiate, a process that starts with a fertilized egg and culminates in the consummate complexity of an adult organism. Even more important in the short run, this knowledge makes possible attempts to treat the many diseases that can arise when immune cells either fail to develop normally in the fetus or deviate from their proper pattern of growth later in life.

The current understanding of how the various components of the immune system develop is almost completely at odds with beliefs that researchers held only three decades ago. We now know that all immune systems derive from a relatively small number of progenitors in the bone marrow and thymus. Before the 1960s, immunologists thought all the different kinds of cells required for an immune response were produced locally in lymphoid organs such as the spleen, appendix and lymph nodes, which are distributed throughout the body. That view began to change as a result of animal experiments and clinical observations of immune system dysfunction.

Perhaps the earliest of the pivotal events leading to the modern theories of immune cell origin were the atomic bomb attacks on Hiroshima and Nagasaki. Many people exposed to radiation released by the explosions died 10 to 15 days later from internal

Figure 2.1 *B* LYMPHOCYTE prepares to enter a blood vessel and leave the bone marrow, where it was produced. Immune cells mature in the thymus and in the bone marrow, then circulate through the body and lymphoid organs such as the spleen and lymph nodes.

bleeding or infection. Animal experiments conducted to explore what happened to such casualties revealed that whole-body radiation kills the generative cells in blood-forming and lymphoid organs. Without the cells responsible for clotting and for fighting invaders, the body dies.

Investigators found that the radiation syndrome could be treated by injecting a small sample of bone marrow cells from a genetically identical donor. Further work with mice demonstrated that the entire blood and immune systems of mice that recovered from radiation were derived from donor cells. A fraction of the newly reconstituted bone marrow from these irradiated mice could in turn save other mice exposed to radiation. Clearly, the bone marrow contained cells capable both of differentiating into all blood cell lineages and of reproducing themselves.

Immunologists discovered fairly early that some bone marrow cells can give rise to progeny of several different types—but not necessarily all. These parents can be defined by their individual characteristics and by the characteristics of their lineages (all cells arising from one precursor are said to belong to a single clone). Workers can grow cells from many different clones in culture to provide enough cells at each stage of differentiation for analysis.

In 1961 Ernest A. McCulloch and James E. Till of the Ontario Cancer Institute in Toronto found evidence that a single cell of the proper kind could in theory reconstitute an entire blood system. They injected bone marrow cells into irradiated mice and noticed that many of the mice developed bumps on their spleens. Each bump contained several distinct cell types. The two workers and their colleagues showed that all the cells in a bump were derived from a single progenitor. They proposed the existence of a relatively rare population of cells—hematopoietic stem cells—that could both reproduce themselves and also generate all blood cell types.

The establishment of the crucial part played by bone marrow cells was followed by discovery of a similarly essential role for the thymus. Removal of the thymus from newborn mice compromised the development of lymphocytes elsewhere in the body. (Lymphocytes are white blood cells that attack bacteria and other foreign matter.) The mice from which the thymus had been removed experienced severe lifelong immunodeficiency.

In another important group of experiments, researchers removed a lymphoid organ called the bursa of Fabricius from chicks (the bursa plays the role in chickens that bone marrow does in humans). That operation did not affect the same lymphocyte lineages that removal of the thymus did; instead it stopped production of cells that matured to become plasma cells, which secrete antibodies. The chicks thus exhibited immunodeficiency of a different kind.

Clinical observations provided complementary evidence for the existence of two lymphoid lineages. In some infants the thymus developed normally, but the bone marrow malfunctioned. These children had lymphocytes in their peripheral tissues but suffered from a congenital deficiency of plasma cells. Conversely, infants born without a thymus but with normal bone marrow produced plasma cells but only a small number of lymphocytes.

Studies of lymphoid malignancies revealed the same developmental pattern. Many kinds of lymphoid tumors in mice were found to originate in the thymus, and early removal of the organ prevented the development of lymphomas elsewhere. Meanwhile a different lymphoma in chickens could be cured by removing the bursa of Fabricius. Apparently, the two lymphoid organs have distinct, essential functions. Each seems responsible for a different class of immune cell.

By the late 1960s, it had become clear that stem cells give rise to two broad lineages of lymphocytes (as well as the other blood cells). One consists of the B cells, which originate in the bone marrow and produce antibodies that bind to foreign proteins and mark them for attack by other cells (see Figure 2.1). They act against extracellular pathogens such as bacteria. The other, the T cells, arises in the thymus (see Figure 2.2). T cells handle such intracellular pathogens as viruses in addition to such intracellular parasites as tuberculosis. T cells also secrete molecules known as lymphokines, which direct the activity of B cells, other T cells and other parts of the immune system.

Once formed, cells of both types migrate to the spleen, lymph nodes and intestinal lymphoid tissues. There they can encounter antigen, the molecular signature of microbial or viral invaders, and be called into action. Lymphocytes continuously circulate through the body's vascular and lymphatic systems, stopping periodically in the lymphoid organs as they patrol for foreign antigens.

Although the existence of the stem cell was first posited in 1961, researchers made little

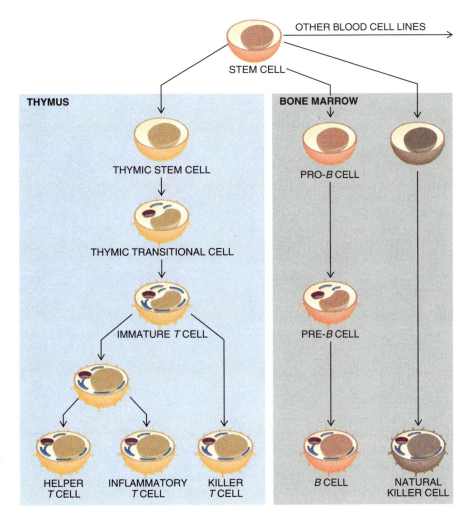

Figure 2.2 CELL LINEAGES of immune and blood cells all begin with the stem cell. Stem cells that differentiate to generate *B* cells reside in the bone marrow, and those that produce *T* cells reside in the thymus.

progress in identifying actual examples until the early 1980s. At that time, biologists established specific assays for *B*, *T* and myeloid precursors. They could then isolate bone marrow cells to determine which surface proteins were present or absent on particular clone-forming cells. In mice, scientists in one of our laboratories (Weissman's) found progenitors for *B*, *T* and other blood cells in only a small fraction of the total population of bone marrow cells, about one in 2,000. These turned out to be stem cells.

The search for human stem cells required the same kinds of techniques that had proved so useful

in mice. In the course of this search, Joseph M. McCune and his colleagues at Stanford University developed a technique that turned out to allow the testing of this fraction of bone marrow cells to determine whether it contained true stem cells that could reproduce themselves. McCune and his colleagues implanted human fetal thymus, liver, bone marrow and lymph nodes into a strain of mice that had no immune system of their own. They succeeded in establishing a functioning human blood-forming and *T* cell–developing system. Since doing this work, McCune has founded a biotechnology company, SyStemix (with which Weissman is associated).

Researchers at SyStemix injected candidate human stem cells into these mice and showed that they could thereby reconstitute the blood-forming and immune systems. Interestingly, the human-derived thymus cells also proved vulnerable to infection with the human immunodeficiency virus (HIV), which causes AIDS; the infection depleted the same kind of circulating human immune cells that are destroyed in AIDS.

Stem cells differentiate into B or T lineages in response to cues (many of them still unknown) from their environment. This phenomenon can be seen in the embryo, where the distinction between B and T cells becomes clear. Early in fetal life, stem cells migrate from the blood-forming organs to the thymus in distinct waves. Once in the thymus, these cohorts of stem cells divide and differentiate. They give rise to successive kinds of T cells that populate the lining (epithelium) of the skin, various orifices (such as the mouth and vagina) and the organs that connect with them (the gastrointestinal tract, uterus and so forth) before producing the later generations that circulate to the lymphoid organs.

These cells can be distinguished by the molecules (known as TCRs, for T cell receptors) they carry on their surface. Moreover, they appear to be produced in a very specific order. Early cells carry receptors whose components consist of so-called gamma and delta chains, whereas later ones carry receptors made of alpha and beta chains.

In mice, for example, the first wave of cells appears between the 13th and 15th days of gestation and carries a TCR type known as gamma 3. These cells emigrate to the skin, where they may serve as sentinels that recognize and destroy skin cells that have become infected, cancerous or otherwise damaged.

The next wave, which appears between the 15th and 20th days of gestation, takes up residence mainly in the lining of the reproductive organs in females and in the epithelium of the tongue in both sexes. These cells carry a TCR called gamma 4. Subsequent waves emigrate for the most part to the spleen (gamma 2) and to the lining of the intestinal tract (gamma 5).

The first and second waves of these cells are made only in the fetal thymus. Later in development and throughout life, the stem cells that settle in the thymus differentiate predominantly into T cells carrying alpha-beta receptors, the so-called helper and killer T cells.

The order in which stem cells generate these waves of progeny matches the order in which DNA encoding the different gamma-chain types appears on the TCR gene. It appears that the stem cells "read out" a development program that depends on the age of the animal.

Early development of the B cell system proceeds along similar but less complex lines. The stem cell progeny that enter the B cell path do so in the same tissues in which other white blood and red blood cells are formed. Early in embryonic life they are produced in the liver, but later the stem cells migrate to the bone marrow.

B cells generated in the fetal liver may differ from those formed later in the bone marrow. The earlier cells make antibodies that can bind to a wide variety of antigens but with relatively low affinity. The later cells, in contrast, carry antibodies that react much more strongly but with only one or two antigens. It appears that the mechanisms that B cells employ to produce a full range of antibodies come into play only near the time of birth. Each B cell in the mature organism bears on its surface a unique antibody receptor complex that it uses to recognize a specific antigen.

Scientists have learned a great deal about how a few stem cells can produce this enormous diversity of B cells. To trace the process, experimenters have learned to recognize the many surface proteins that cells express as they divide and progress along the B cell path of differentiation. These molecular markers are a primary means by which cells interact with nearby cells; consequently, a B lymphocyte will display different proteins as it matures.

The signals that tell a stem cell daughter to enter the B cell pathway instead of becoming a red cell or another type of white cell appear to come primarily from other cells in the immediate environment. When the late Cheryl Whitlock and Owen N. Witte of the University of California at Los Angeles first discovered how to raise B cells in long-term cultures, they found that stromal cells (large, veil-like cells in the bone marrow) are essential for culturing B cells. The stromal cells interact with progenitor B (pro-B) cells by means of surface molecules. They also make soluble protein factors (such as interleukin-7) that bind to receptors on the pro-B and pre-B cells, signaling them to divide and to differentiate (see Figure 2.3).

As they divide, pro-B cells begin the process that will culminate in the expression of a unique antibody receptor complex. First, they rearrange the

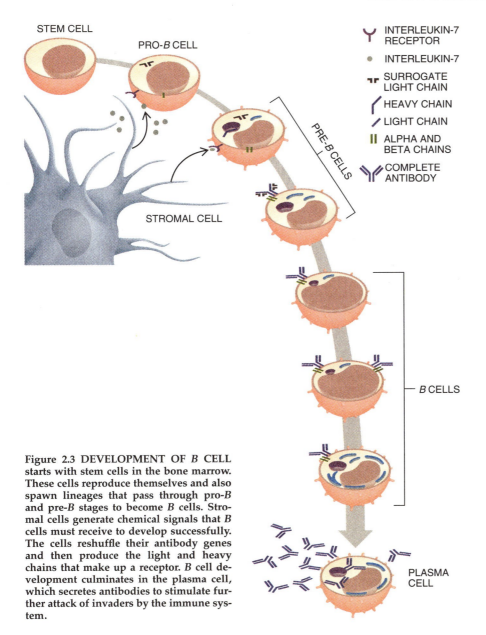

STEM CELL

PRO-*B* CELL

STROMAL CELL

PRE-*B* CELLS

INTERLEUKIN-7
RECEPTOR

INTERLEUKIN-7

SURROGATE
LIGHT CHAIN

HEAVY CHAIN

LIGHT CHAIN

ALPHA AND
BETA CHAINS

COMPLETE
ANTIBODY

B CELLS

PLASMA
CELL

Figure 2.3 DEVELOPMENT OF *B* CELL starts with stem cells in the bone marrow. These cells reproduce themselves and also spawn lineages that pass through pro-*B* and pre-*B* stages to become *B* cells. Stromal cells generate chemical signals that *B* cells must receive to develop successfully. The cells reshuffle their antibody genes and then produce the light and heavy chains that make up a receptor. *B* cell development culminates in the plasma cell, which secretes antibodies to stimulate further attack of invaders by the immune system.

gene fragments that encode the light and heavy immunoglobulin chains that will form an antibody molecule. These genes are actively transcribed as soon as rearrangement is complete.

The order in which the gene fragments begin functioning is crucial to the later development of the *B* cell. The genes directing the construction of the heavy chains are typically shuffled and begin functioning first. (The cells are then called pre-*B*

cells.) The genes encoding light chains are then rearranged and also start functioning (see Chapter 3, "How the Immune System Recognizes Invaders," by Charles A. Janeway, Jr.).

These cells also commence to produce two additional proteins, immunoglobulins alpha and beta (Ig alpha and beta), which span cell membranes. The immunoglobulin heavy chains and their light-chain partners associate with Ig alpha and Ig beta to form an antigen receptor unit that migrates to the cell surface. There it can interact with antigens and send appropriate signals back to the nucleus. Cells that reach this stage of differentiation are called B cells, and they enter the bloodstream en route to peripheral tissues.

The B cell population can respond to an extremely diverse range of antigens. To guide the manufacture of its light and heavy chains, each cell selects one combination of its gene fragments out of more than a million possibilities. In addition, each developing cell can modify the gene-splicing sites to further increase variability in the DNA encoding the antigen-binding site. And—as if that diversity were still insufficient—the cell can even insert new nucleotide sequences at the joint between fragments as it splices them together.

The cell rewrites its genetic code by means of the enzyme terminal deoxynucleotide transferase. This enzyme is expressed only in the nucleus of pro-B cells, where heavy-chain gene rearrangement usually occurs. Sometimes, however, light-chain genes are rearranged first. Hiromi Kubagawa of the University of Alabama at Birmingham uncovered this fact when he infected early B lineage cells with Epstein-Barr virus, creating a self-reproducing culture whose immunoglobulin genes were frozen at that early stage of development. He found pre-B cells that had rearranged only their light chains; their joints contained new sequences, suggesting that the shuffling had taken place before transferase activity stopped.

Thus far we have been discussing B cell development as if it were a path that all cells follow to the end once they have embarked on it. That is not the case. When Dennis G. Osmond, now at McGill University, counted the number of cells in the pro-B, pre-B and B stages in mouse bone marrow, he found that half or more of the cells apparently die during the pre-B stage.

Researchers theorize that pre-B cells die unless they receive a survival signal—some kind of molecular messenger from nearby cells. The "kiss of life" may bind to a receptor that appears on the surface of late-stage pre-B cells. This receptor is composed of heavy chains paired with a so-called surrogate light-chain complex. The surrogate complex, unlike the antigen receptors produced by mature B cells, is encoded by genes that do not require rearrangement for their expression.

When Daisuke Kitamura and his colleagues at the University of Cologne prevented the expression of these receptors, they found that the production of B cells fell to less than a tenth its normal level. The B cells that survived may have been ones that rearranged their light-chain genes early, thus producing nonsurrogate light chains at an early enough stage to substitute for the missing receptor.

Other B cells die not because they fail to receive a kiss of life but rather because they carry a kiss of death. Some rearrangements of a B cell's gene fragments will make antibodies that react to the body's own cells. Lineages carrying these antibodies must be eliminated.

The negative selection process begins when newly formed B cells first interact with their environment. Self-reactive cells rapidly encounter large quantities of antigen to which their antibodies can bind—molecules on the surfaces of their neighbors. If the binding is strong enough, the antibody receptor will transmit signals into the cell, causing it to commit suicide in what is known as apoptosis (programmed cell death). Immature B cells that do not react strongly to self-antigen survive and mature. Later they can respond to antigenic stimulation from nonself molecules. This general principle was first demonstrated in chicks and mice treated with antibodies against the IgM receptors on immature B cells: early administration of receptor antibodies aborted B cell development, whereas doses given later stimulated it. Early in development the signal transmitted by the antibody receptors induces apoptosis by activating enzymes that cleave nuclear DNA. Virtually no reactive B cells survive to maturity.

Clones that survive the selection process can migrate to the peripheral lymphoid tissues. There they finally begin the working phase of their life history. Eventually, after being stimulated by both antigens and T cells, they may return to the bone marrow to undertake their final maturation into antibody-secreting plasma cells.

The T cell pathway is somewhat more complex. Stem cells in the thymus that commit to this line of development may eventually mature into several different kinds of T cells, including helper and killer.

Developing T cells pass through a number of winnowing points. The first challenge tests their ability to recognize antigens presented to them by other cells—an essential attribute for a functioning immune cell. Molecules of the so-called major histocompatibility complex (MHC) hold fragments of protein antigens for presentation to *T* cells. MHC molecules are divided into two types, class I and class II. Developing cells in the thymus scan their environment to determine whether they recognize any self-MHC. If they can, they survive; if not, they die (see Figure 2.4).

Once the maturing *T* cells have survived this challenge, the next step is the destruction of the cells bearing receptors that react too well to the body's own tissues (just as with *B* cells). Ultimately, only *T* cells with receptors that can recognize both foreign peptides and self-MHC survive to leave the thymus and take up residence throughout the body.

Immunologists trying to fill in the details of this picture started by tracing the line of descent from stem cell to emigrant *T* cell. To test lineage relationships, researchers used stem cells and progeny bearing clearly recognizable markers. They introduced these cells, at different stages of maturation, into the thymuses of mice whose cells bore no such markers. By waiting hours or days, the workers could then determine what offspring their transplants had spawned.

Thymic cells transplanted at the earliest stage of development express virtually none of the common *T* cell markers on their surfaces: little or no CD4 co-receptor protein and neither *T* cell receptor structures nor the co-receptor protein known as CD8. (CD8 binds to class I MHC, whereas CD4 binds to

class II MHC.) A day after transplantation, however, these large cells have reproduced themselves and given rise to other large cells bearing CD8 but no CD4 or TCR (human thymic cells at a similar stage of development express CD4 but not CD8 or TCR). These cells in turn divide into progeny that bear CD4, CD8 and small amounts of TCR. This stage is the first at which a *T* cell progenitor expresses TCR on its surface. The expression of CD4 at these early stages of development may explain why HIV so virulently depletes *T* cells: the virus is believed to bind to CD4 molecules, and so it may attack these primitive thymic progenitors, cutting off the entire line of their progeny (see Chapter 6, "AIDS and the Immune System," by Warner C. Greene).

While the cells are dividing and changing their surface proteins, they are also rearranging their genes to produce *T* cell receptors. In the mouse, for example, assembly and surface expression of TCR chains begin at or before the stage at which they express both CD4 and CD8. These progenitors are poised to interact with MHC-bearing cells in the thymus. Most of those binding to class I MHC molecules will become killer cells. Those binding to class II develop mainly into helper cells, although some also become killer cells. (Cells that do not bind to any MHC shrink and die.)

Once they have become committed to one path, the intermediate-stage cells shut down production of the receptor type they will no longer use (either CD8 or CD4) and express additional TCR. They

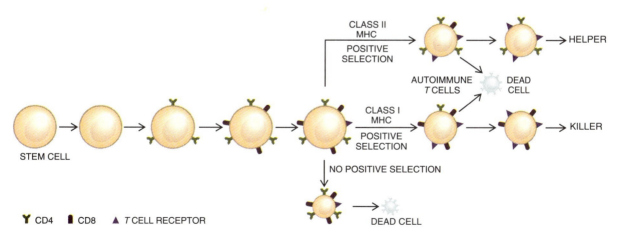

CLASS II MHC POSITIVE SELECTION → HELPER

AUTOIMMUNE *T* CELLS — DEAD CELL

STEM CELL

CLASS I MHC POSITIVE SELECTION → KILLER

NO POSITIVE SELECTION

DEAD CELL

Ⓨ CD4   ▮ CD8   ▲ *T* CELL RECEPTOR

Figure 2.4 *T* CELLS are produced in the thymus by stem cells that have migrated from the bone marrow. The maturing cells go through stages that can be distinguished by the surface proteins they express. Those whose receptors bind to class II MHC molecules on adjacent cells will eventually become so-called helper *T* cells, and those whose receptors bind to class I MHC molecules will for the most part become killer *T* cells. (MHC is a molecule that cells use to present antigens to *T* cells.) Those that do not bind to any MHC or that bind to the body's own antigens will die.

also acquire "homing receptors" that enable them to leave the bloodstream and enter the peripheral lymphoid organs. Finally, they leave the thymus.

Not all potential *T* cells, of course, complete this line of development. Some undergo negative selection, in which signals from other cells (those carrying self-antigen attached to self-MHC) cause apoptosis. Cells in the thymus can supposedly trigger positive or negative selection depending on the layer of primitive fetal tissue from which they derived: endoderm, mesoderm or ectoderm. The thymus is unusual among lymphoid organs in containing cells from all three sources.

At this point, the cellular pathways that diverged when particular stem cells began differentiating into *B* or *T* cells come together in the peripheral tissues. Most of the remaining stages in the development of both kinds of cells take place once their receptors have been triggered by encounters with a foreign substance.

Inside the lymphoid organs, *T* and *B* cells that have matured but are not yet engaged in immune responses reside in separate domains. After immune cells have been stimulated by antigens, the cells that will participate in antibody production undergo a complex set of interactions to form new structures called germinal centers.

Three kinds of cells congregate in these germinal centers at the interface between *T* and *B* domains: activated helper *T* cells, *B* cells and dendritic cells, a type of antigen-presenting cell. A few *B* cells proliferate in response to the antigen; soon their clones make up most of the population in the centers.

While they are proliferating, the *B* cells also differentiate and mutate. They modify the DNA in their gene fragments to make antibodies similar to those that bound to the antigen in question (but perhaps even more reactive). Some of the *B* cells interact with helper *T* cells and then give rise to plasma cells. There are several kinds of plasma cells; the antibodies they generate all react to the same antigen but elicit different immune responses. Yet other *B* cells become so-called memory cells. They will not participate immediately in the body's defense but rather will retain a molecular record of past invaders to speed response in the future (see Figure 2.5).

Although the immune response is orchestrated within the lymphoid organs, lymphocytes do not merely reside there waiting to be called on. James L. Gowans and his colleagues at the University of Oxford demonstrated in 1959 that immune cells circulate between the bloodstream and the lymphoid organs. This traffic provides each lymphoid organ with a rapid sampling of all lymphocytes that might possess receptors for the foreign antigens currently attracting the body's attention.

Circulating lymphocytes pass into lymphoid organs by means of a specialized kind of blood vessel, the HEV (high endothelial venule, named for the blocky surface of its walls). Only lymphocytes can pass through the HEVs; they express homing receptors that match counter receptors on the HEV walls. These receptors appear to come in two varieties: one that homes in on lymph nodes, and another that matches surface molecules expressed by lymphoid organs in the gastrointestinal tract.

When *T* and *B* cells are activated, they quickly stop producing their usual homing receptor molecules and revert to making another integrin that they produced early in their development. This molecule binds to the vascular-cell adhesion molecule, VCAM-1 (which also appears on stromal cells in the bone marrow and epithelial cells inside the thymus). As a result, these activated cells no longer pass through the walls of normal lymphoid-organ HEVs when they are released into the bloodstream. Instead they home in on blood vessels serving infected, inflamed and antigen-bearing tissues (see Figure 2.6). The vessels in these inflamed areas may express VCAM-1, whereas those elsewhere do not. By returning to a cellular expression of their early development, the cells fulfill their ultimate task.

This simplified version of how the cells of the immune system develop and mature does not tell the entire story. For example, a number of other adhesion molecules are involved in interactions between lymphocytes and endothelial or stromal cells. Indeed, researchers still have much to learn about the means by which cells receive the signals that cause them to undergo programmed death, to continue living or to grow and differentiate.

One important question is how stem cells choose between reproducing themselves and producing offspring committed to a particular lineage. This problem is of more than theoretical significance: if stem cells prove useful in the restoration of congenital or acquired immunodeficiencies, methods that increase their numbers either in the test tube or in the body might improve patients' chances for recovery. Stem cells are also an obvious target for gene therapy that might either replace a defective gene or endow the

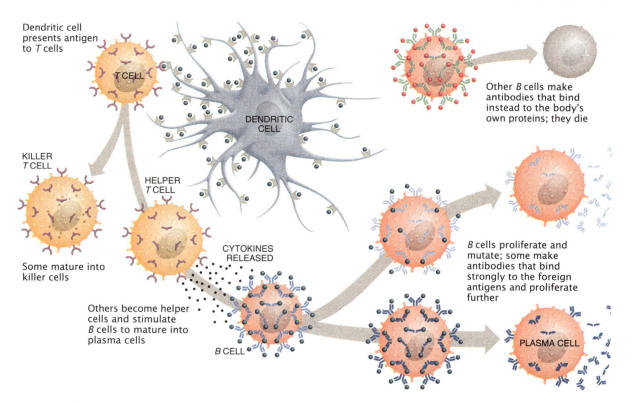

Dendritic cell presents antigen to T cells

T CELL

DENDRITIC CELL

KILLER T CELL

HELPER T CELL

Some mature into killer cells

CYTOKINES RELEASED

Others become helper cells and stimulate B cells to mature into plasma cells

B CELL

Other B cells make antibodies that bind instead to the body's own proteins; they die

B cells proliferate and mutate; some make antibodies that bind strongly to the foreign antigens and proliferate further

PLASMA CELL

Figure 2.5 IMMUNE RESPONSE takes place in lymph nodes, where T and B cells congregate. Dendritic cells present antigen to T cells (center). These T cells, called helper-cells, interact with other T and B cells to produce both killer T cells (left) that leave the lymph node in search of infected tissue and plasma cells (right) that secrete antibodies.

cells' progeny with abilities to survive in a hostile environment, such as a body carrying HIV.

In addition, as researchers understand more fully the path from stem cell to activated B or T cells, they will make headway in treating diseases where that development goes dangerously wrong. Inherited or acquired defects in genes essential for the growth and differentiation of immunocompetent cells can result in immunodeficiency or lymphoid malignancies.

Inherited defects can block development of T or B cells at many different stages, depending on the product of the gene in question. For example, a defect in the gene encoding the enzyme adenosine deaminase (ADA) allows toxic metabolic products to accumulate in the bone marrow and thymus, preventing lymphocytes from synthesizing DNA and dividing. Affected infants lack T and B cells and so cannot defend themselves against infection (hence the term "severe combined immunodeficiency disease," or SCID). Armed with an understanding of the function of stem cells, Robert A. Good and his colleagues at the University of Minnesota Medical School showed that SCID could be cured by transplanting compatible bone marrow from a healthy sibling, but unfortunately most patients lack a suitable donor. Michael R. Blaese and his co-workers at the National Cancer Institute, however, have succeeded in inserting a functional ADA gene in deficient T lymphocytes, thereby repairing one essential limb of the immune system.

During the first half of 1993, researchers found the genes responsible for three other immunodeficiency diseases. All are on the X chromosome and affect boys (who have only one copy of the X's genetic information), but each aborts immune system development at a different level. One, a mutation in a protein kinase gene essential for transmitting signals for pre-B cell growth and development, causes a gross deficit of mature B cells and the

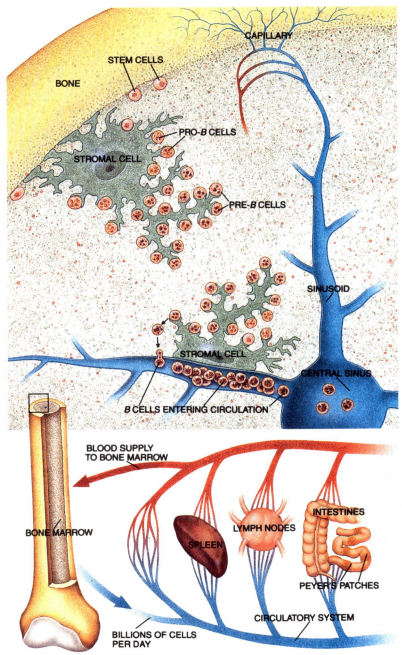

Figure 2.6 IMMUNE SYSTEM CIRCU-LATION commences in the bone marrow, where *B* cells mature (*top*). Cells leaving the marrow (*bottom*) take up residence in the spleen, lymph nodes and Peyer's patches of the intestines. *B* and *T* cells circulate continuously through the body, patrolling for antigens that could signal infection.

antibodies they secrete. Another is the consequence of a mutation in the gene for one of the three chains that make up the receptor for the growth factor inter-leukin-2. This defect sabotages the development of helper *T* cells, which in turn prevents *B* cells from maturing into plasma cells. The third disorder to be

elucidated is caused by a defect in the gene encoding the surface molecules through which *T* and *B* cells interact. Boys in whom the CD40 molecule or its receptor is malformed produce only IgM antibodies; they lack the signal that causes *B* cells to divide and make high-affinity antibodies of other classes.

Identification of these genes could lead to gene replacement therapy for these deficiencies. These three gene defects were discovered almost simultaneously by several groups of investigators; knowledge of the development and function of the immune system may have reached a level at which the genetic basis for other immune disorders may soon also be found. Consequently, clinical benefits may accrue rapidly.

Although lymphoid malignancies also result from genetic malfunctions, they differ in a number of ways from immunodeficiency diseases. Most important, malignancy requires the accumulation of several mutations, all of which favor excessive cell growth and survival at the expense of maturation and natural death. Complex multicellular organisms have evolved many checkpoints for monitoring cell growth and survival.

To overcome this complex defense, the malignant sequence of mutations must usually begin in the stem cells or their immediate clonal progeny to permit the gradual evolution of a malignant clone of cells that can elude all these monitoring mechanisms. Even if a person inherits a gene predisposing to malignancy, the affected cells must acquire additional mutations during their life span to become malignant. Once one mutation favoring growth or survival occurs, however, the odds increase that a cell will persist long enough to suffer another growth-promoting mutation and thus a third or fourth.

This principle can be seen in follicular lymphoma, an extremely slow growing malignancy of *B* cells in germinal centers. Virtually all follicular lymphomas contain a translocation of a gene called *bcl-2*, which produces a messenger that prevents programmed cell death. The gene is usually turned off when an activated *B* cell fails to recognize antigen or reshuffles its mini-genes so as to make self-reacting antibodies, but in follicular lymphoma cells it resides next to an antibody gene that is turned on in *B* cells and so remains active indefinitely.

The multistep path to malignancy may also explain why *B* cell malignancies are four times as common as those involving *T* cells. Stem cells in the bone marrow produce *B* cells throughout life (and thus have many years over which to accumulate mutations). Most *T* cells, in contrast, are produced early in life; the thymus withers as people age, leaving fewer thymic stem cells and their offspring to mutate.

Once developmental and molecular biologists unravel the signals that guide stem cells and their intricate lines of progeny, they may be able to manipulate the development of the immune system from without. Clinicians will then be able to strengthen responses to invaders, mitigate the damage that immune cells do to self, and correct or eliminate those cell lines that would otherwise propagate families of malignancy.

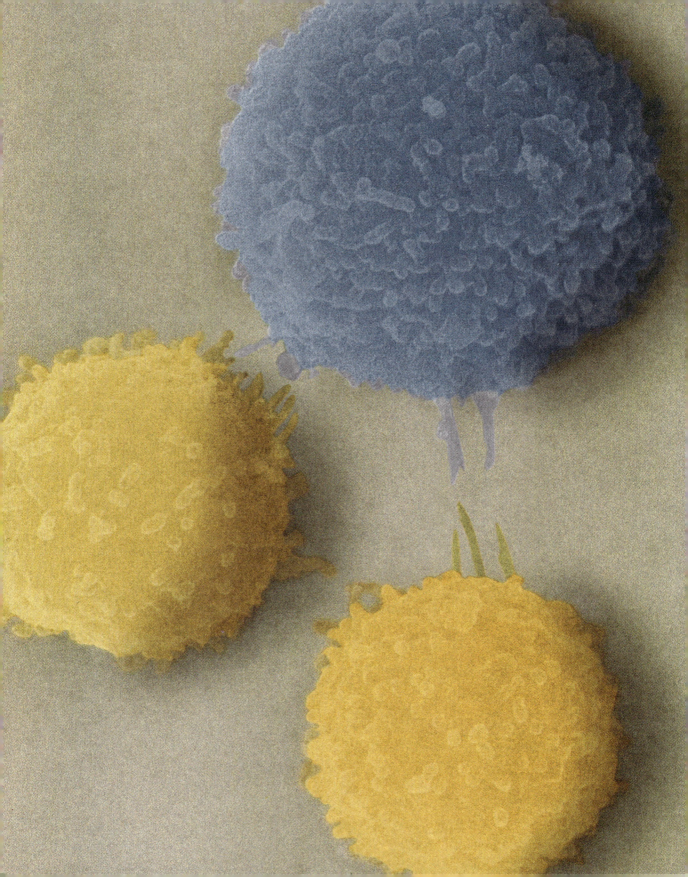

How the Immune System Recognizes Invaders

Cells of the immune system recombine gene fragments to create the millions of receptors needed to identify and attack the myriad pathogens encountered throughout life.

· · ·

Charles A. Janeway, Jr.

Thirty-six years ago an article entitled "Agammaglobulinemia" appeared in SCIENTIFIC AMERICAN. One of the authors was my father. In the piece, he described an illness resulting from a defect in the body's defenses against infection, a failure in the immune system's mechanism for detecting pathogens. His work and that of Ogden Bruton in identifying the first known immunodeficiency disease helped to break a path that has led to a deep and useful understanding of how the immune system recognizes and distinguishes the molecules of the body from those of an invading bacterium, virus or parasite.

People who have agammaglobulinemia cannot make antibody molecules. These specialized proteins, found in the blood and extracellular fluid, normally bind to the bacteria or viruses that cause infections and serve as a signal to the attacking molecules and cells of the immune system. The ability of molecules such as antibodies to identify foreign molecules and so to guide the body's defenses confers important advantages. It enables us to eliminate infections, to resist reinfection and to be protected by vaccination.

Some of these same mechanisms, unfortunately, can trigger disease instead of controlling it. The immune system might, for example, react to a harmless foreign substance, such as pollen, producing allergy. Events can take a more serious turn when an immune attack focuses on the body's own tissues, leading to an autoimmune disease. But whether they contribute to health or to disease, the mechanisms of recognition and response are the same. Recognition mechanisms are therefore crucial to understanding how the immune system works and how it fails.

In this chapter, I describe the two main systems by which the body identifies foreign material. The first is the innate immune system—innate in the sense that the body is born with the ability to recognize certain microbes immediately and to destroy them. The second is the adaptive immune system, in which antibodies play a leading role. The receptors used in the adaptive immune response are formed by piecing together gene segments, like a patchwork quilt. Each cell uses the available pieces differently to make a unique receptor, enabling the cells collectively to recognize the infectious organisms confronted during a

Figure 3.1 T CELLS (*yellow*), a kind of lymphocyte, use special receptors on their surface to detect an infected macrophage (*blue*). These T cells represent only part of the repertoire the immune system has to recognize pathogens.

lifetime. Understanding the genes, molecules and cells that make up the immune system has enabled researchers to determine the etiology of diseases, including agammaglobulinemia, and to start work on cures.

Our innate immune system can destroy many pathogens on first encounter. An important component of the innate response is a class of blood proteins known as complement. Their name comes from their ability to assist, or complement the activity of, antibodies in fighting infection. Discovered by the Belgian bacteriologist Jules Bordet in 1900, complement can act in many ways (see Figure 3.2). One type of complement protein, when chemically stimulated, can bind to any protein—those on bacteria as well as those on our own cells. The bound protein triggers the activity of the other complement molecules. These bound molecules attract phagocytes, amoebalike cells that engulf and digest microbes wearing a complement coat. Complement can also kill cells and bacteria by punching pores in their lipid membrane. The holes allow water to rush in, a process that destroys the cell. Complement protects against such diseases as bacterial meningitis and gonorrhea.

Yet this powerful attack system does not destroy our own cells. Unlike microbes, our cells are equipped with proteins that inactivate complement. Thus, at this simplest of levels, innate immunity distinguishes the molecules that make up the body, called self, from all other molecules, or nonself.

Not all pathogens are so easily disposed of by the complement system. Some have devised ways of avoiding attack by complement. The bacteria that cause pneumonia and strep throat have capsules, coats made up of long chains of sugar molecules (polysaccharides). These capsules prevent complement from acting directly on the bacteria.

The innate immune system has two ways of coping with these types of bacteria. First, throughout the tissues of the body are the large phagocytes called macrophages. Macrophages have receptors for some of these polysaccharides, and they use these receptors to bind to and ingest bacteria. Second, macrophages that meet bacteria can secrete interleukin-6, a protein that in turn stimulates the liver. Interleukin-6 instructs the liver to secrete a new protein, one that binds to sugar residues called mannose. These residues protrude from the bacterial capsule. After this mannose-binding protein binds to the bacteria, it changes its shape so that it activates the complement cascade and turns on phagocytes. In this way, mannose-binding protein tells the body which particles must be bound.

Innate immunity, however, cannot protect against all infections. Microbes evolve rapidly, enabling them to devise means to evade the inherited immune defenses of humans and other species that evolve more slowly. To compensate, vertebrates have a unique strategy of immune recognition: adaptive immunity. Adaptive immunity enables the body to recognize and to respond to any microbe, even if it has never faced the invader before.

Adaptive immunity operates by the process of clonal selection, an idea formulated in the 1950s by Sir Frank Macfarlane Burnet of the Walter and Eliza Hall Institute of Medical Research in Australia and now widely accepted. In clonal selection, cells of the adaptive immune system, known as B lymphocytes, or B cells for short, manufacture antibodies and display them on the cell surface. The antibody then serves as a receptor. Each B cell makes a different receptor, so that each recognizes a different foreign molecule. Armed with these receptors, the B cells act as sentries, always on the lookout for microbes. If a B cell finds such an intruder, it divides rapidly. Because all the daughter cells come from one parent, they are known as a clone (hence the term "clonal selection"). All the cells in each clone have the same receptor. These cloned B cells then differentiate into cells that secrete antibodies, which, like the B cell receptor, bind to the microbes. Once flagged as foreign by the antibodies, the microbes are removed from the body by phagocytes and by the complement system.

A critical question in understanding adaptive immunity is how B lymphocytes generate so many different receptors. More specifically, how could the millions of different receptors necessary to recognize all microbes be encoded in a limited genome? A person has only about 100,000 genes, but the 10 trillion B cells in an individual can make more than 100 million distinct antibody proteins at any one time. We obviously cannot inherit the genes necessary to specify all these proteins.

The answer was discovered in recent years, as investigators identified the genes that encode antibodies and B cell receptors. One key was discov-

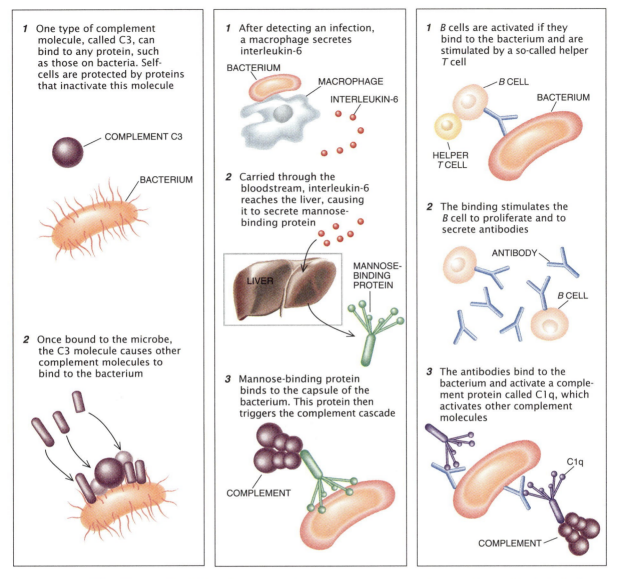

1 One type of complement molecule, called C3, can bind to any protein, such as those on bacteria. Self-cells are protected by proteins that inactivate this molecule

COMPLEMENT C3

BACTERIUM

2 Once bound to the microbe, the C3 molecule causes other complement molecules to bind to the bacterium

1 After detecting an infection, a macrophage secretes interleukin-6

BACTERIUM

MACROPHAGE

INTERLEUKIN-6

2 Carried through the bloodstream, interleukin-6 reaches the liver, causing it to secrete mannose-binding protein

LIVER

MANNOSE-BINDING PROTEIN

3 Mannose-binding protein binds to the capsule of the bacterium. This protein then triggers the complement cascade

COMPLEMENT

1 B cells are activated if they bind to the bacterium and are stimulated by a so-called helper T cell

B CELL

BACTERIUM

HELPER T CELL

2 The binding stimulates the B cell to proliferate and to secrete antibodies

ANTIBODY

B CELL

3 The antibodies bind to the bacterium and activate a complement protein called C1q, which activates other complement molecules

C1q

COMPLEMENT

Figure 3.2 COMPLEMENT ACTIVITY can be triggered in three ways. Complement can act directly on bacteria (*left*), or it can be activated by mannose-binding protein (*center*). Antibodies produced as a result of infection can also acti-vate complement (*right*). Complement then kills the bacteria or recruits other immune system cells, such as phago-cytes.

ered in 1976 by Susumu Tonegawa, then working at the Basel Institute for Immunology. He showed that antibody genes are inherited as gene frag-ments. These fragments are joined together to form a complete gene only in individual lympho-cytes as they develop.

The joining process itself generates still more di-

versity. In 1980 Fred Alt and David Baltimore of the Massachusetts Institute of Technology showed that the enzymes that combine gene segments add random DNA bases to the ends of the pieces being joined. As a result, new genes, each encoding a protein chain, are formed. Further diversity re-sults from the assembly of protein chains into a complete receptor. Antibodies are made from two pairs of protein chains: a heavy chain and a light chain. The heavy chains are connected to form a Y, with the light chains located on the upper branches, alongside the heavy chains. Each *B* cell produces just one kind of light chain and one kind of heavy chain, so that each *B* cell makes a unique antibody receptor (see Figure 3.3). In fact, 1,000 different chains of each type can in theory form a million combinations. All these random joining processes can create more distinct antibody molecules than there are *B* cells in the body.

As if these processes did not generate sufficient diversity, the genes for receptors of *B* lymphocytes mutate extremely rapidly when the *B* cell is activated by binding to a foreign substance or antigen. These "hypermutations" create additional receptors. In effect, the immune system is constantly experimenting with slight variations on successful receptors in pursuit of an optimal immune response.

Once a *B* lymphocyte binds antigen to its receptor, it differentiates and secretes antibody molecules—a soluble form of the receptor—into the

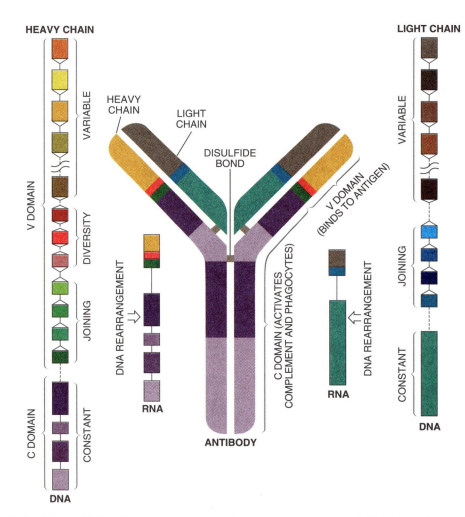

Figure 3.3 ANTIBODY MOLECULE is made up of a pair of heavy chains and a pair of light chains. The chains are encoded by genes that consist of different DNA segments. These segments rearrange to make genes for chains that are different in each *B* cell. The joining is variable, so that only a few gene segments generate the estimated 100 million distinct antibodies the body is capable of producing.

plasma, or fluid component, of the blood. Because this new antibody is specified by the genes that created the receptor on the original *B* cell, it has the identical specificity. But a *B* cell and its progeny can produce a different kind of variation on the antibody molecule. It can do this by altering the so-called constant part of the heavy chain, again by rearranging genes. This second type of gene manipulation creates antibodies that go to different places in the body. These antibodies still recognize the same antigens. After binding to a microbe, these antibody types can begin the complement cascade, activate phagocytes or cause allergic reactions.

Adaptive immunity also is the source of immunologic memory. That is, we resist infections we have already experienced far more efficiently and forcefully than we do infections faced for the first time. We have this memory because the body retains lymphocytes that responded in the initial infection. These cells can be rapidly reactivated when the same types of microbes enter the body, and their antibody products prevent a recurrence of the disease. (In contrast, the innate system does not discriminate one microbe from another and so affords neither more nor less protection after an infection.)

The benefits of adaptive immunity are partially offset by two drawbacks. First, it takes more than five days to develop an antibody response, given that the *B* cells need to proliferate and differentiate before they can make antibodies. The body must rely on the innate immune system to hold infections in check during this period. Second, because any large molecule, such as a protein or a polysaccharide, can be recognized by an antibody, the adaptive immune system on occasion makes antibodies against the body's own cells. These antibodies activate complement so efficiently that the system that prevents complement from attacking the body's cells is overwhelmed. Autoimmune disease is the result. The attack on self is normally avoided through tolerance, a process that eliminates self-reactive cells (see Chapter 4, "How the Immune System Recognizes the Body," by Philippa Marrack and John W. Kappler).

Despite these drawbacks, the strategy of rearranging genes in adaptive immunity has put in place an ingenious protection system. How could such an elaborate process emerge in vertebrates, and how did it become the keystone in adaptive immunity? As with all evolutionary issues, this question can be answered only in terms of models and not with certainty. Nevertheless, our knowledge of receptors does suggest a plausible scenario.

An important clue lies in the fact that all immunologic receptors are built from similar blocks of protein. Each block is encoded in a chunk of DNA known as an exon, or coding sequence. Exons are divided by introns, noncoding DNA that is transcribed into RNA and then later removed by the process of RNA splicing. As a result, the coding blocks form a continuous message.

Each protein component of an antibody has a structure called the immunoglobulin fold. This general structure is used in many proteins besides antibodies; it forms a compact domain of protein comprising strands of amino acids that lie side by side. In antibodies, these domains form the heavy and light chains, connected by a couple of sulfur atoms, a disulfide bond.

Immunoglobulin domains are of two types, called V for variable and C for constant. The V domains in antibodies pair to make the site that recognizes antigens. They are followed by pairs of C domains that mediate function in the molecule, such as complement binding. The V domains consist of partial genes: a V gene segment, a J (for joining) segment and sometimes also a D (for diversity) gene segment. The unique variability of V domains results from gene rearrangement, which generates the diversity of receptors in humans.

Some proteins, however, have domains that resemble the V domains of antibodies but are not produced by gene rearrangement. In these proteins, a single exon specifies the entire V domain. An example of one such protein is the CD4 molecule, which plays a role in immune recognition and is also the target of the AIDS virus. Such intact V genes are in fact found in some primitive vertebrate antibody genes as well.

Our rearranging antibody V genes likely evolved from these intact V genes. Gene rearrangement could have arisen when a mobile bit of DNA, called a transposon, was inserted into an intact V exon. This insertion split the V exon. Split genes are inactive; they could manufacture antibodies only once the intervening transposon is removed and the gene segments are joined to reform the intact exon. Just such a removal mechanism exists in our bodies when *B* lymphocytes generate their receptors. Thus, V gene rearrangement does more than generate diversity in antibodies. It is also crucial in forming the genes that encode antibody proteins. Without rearrangement, no protein can be made from these genes.

Gene rearrangement has proved to be such a powerful means of expressing just one of many related genes that at least one pathogen uses it to avoid detection by the immune system. The trypanosome, a protozoan parasite that causes sleeping sickness, has a single protein in its coat against which the infected host makes antibodies. These antibodies eliminate most of the trypanosomes, but a few of the parasites change their coats by rearranging the coat protein gene. These variant trypanosomes escape detection by the first onslaught of antibodies and continue to grow. The host makes antibody to each variant, but new forms keep arising and growing, causing a relapsing pattern of infection. Here, as in the case of immunologic receptors, rearrangement controls gene expression.

So far we have discussed how the innate immune system, which relies on inherited recognition molecules, and the adaptive system, which relies on gene rearrangement to generate novel receptors in lymphocytes, work together to identify microbes. This dual approach is successful only against pathogens in the body's fluids. Many microbes slip inside the body's cells before antibodies can be made. As water-soluble proteins, antibodies can permeate the extracellular fluid and blood, but they cannot venture across the lipid membranes of cells.

Consequently, the immune system has evolved a special mechanism to detect infections within cells. This mechanism acts in two steps. First, it finds a way to signal to the body that certain cells have been infected. Next, it mobilizes cells specifically designed to recognize these infected cells and to eliminate the infection.

The initial step, signaling that a cell is infected, is accomplished by special molecules that deliver pieces of the microbe to the surface of the infected cell. These molecules, which are synthesized in the endoplasmic reticulum of cells, bind to peptides, small fragments of protein that have been degraded inside the cell. After binding to peptides, these transporter molecules migrate to the cell surface.

These transporters are proteins of the major histocompatibility complex (MHC) of genes. They were discovered by the late British geneticist Peter Gorer and by George D. Snell of Jackson Laboratory in Bar Harbor, Me., as the cause of graft rejection; hence their long-winded name, derived from the Greek word for tissues (histo) and the ability to get along (compatibility). These MHC molecules can be divided into two classes, unimaginatively designated class I and class II MHC molecules. Class I molecules are found on almost all types of body cells. Class II molecules appear only on cells involved in an immune response, such as macrophages and B cells.

Although both types of MHC molecules are structurally distinct, studies published in July 1993 by Jerry H. Brown and Don C. Wiley of Harvard University and their colleagues, as well as earlier work by Pamela J. Bjorkman, now at the California Institute of Technology, and her colleagues, showed that they fold into very similar shapes (see Figure 3.4). Each MHC molecule has a deep groove into which a short peptide, or protein fragment, can bind. Because this peptide is not part of the MHC molecule itself, it can vary from one MHC molecule to the next. On healthy cells, all these peptides come from self-proteins. It is the presence of foreign peptides in the MHC groove that tells the immune system that the cell is infected.

The foreign peptide–MHC complexes displayed by an infected cell are recognized by receptors on a distinct type of lymphocyte, the T cell (see Figure 3.1). The structure of the receptor on T cells is basically the same as that of the membrane-bound antibody molecule that acts as the receptor on B cells. But T cell receptors are specialized to recognize only foreign peptide fragments bound by MHC molecules. When a T cell receptor binds to its specific foreign peptide–MHC complex, the T cell can act to cure or to kill the infected cell.

The two different classes of MHC molecules present peptides that arise in different places within cells. Class I molecules bind to peptides that originate from proteins in the cytosolic compartment of a cell. These proteins are digested inside the cell as part of the natural process by which a cell continually renews its protein contents. James Shepherd, working in my laboratory at Yale University, recently showed that the short peptide fragments that result from this process are pumped by a distinct transporter from the cytosol into the endoplasmic reticulum.

Here the class I MHC molecules are synthesized as long chains of amino acids that must fold to

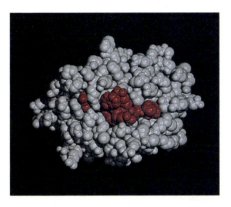
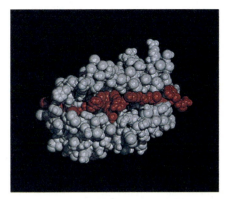

Figure 3.4 **MAJOR HISTOCOMPATIBILITY COMPLEX, or MHC for short, makes two kinds of molecules in cells: class I (*left*) and class II (*right*). The images present the viewpoint of a T cell receptor. Class I MHC molecules can hold** only short peptides (*red*), because the binding site is closed off. In contrast, class II MHC molecules can bind to peptides of different lengths, because the binding site is open at both ends.

yield the mature class I MHC protein. This folding can occur only around a suitable peptide, much as a pearl in an oyster develops around a grain of sand (see boxed figure "Delivering Peptides to the Cell Surface"). The peptides transported there, then, make natural seeds.

The folding of a class I MHC molecule around a peptide signals it to carry the peptide to the surface and hold it there. If the peptide is foreign—stemming from, say, a virus infecting the cell—then a passing T cell will recognize it. The T cells that act in this way are those with CD8 proteins on their surface. These CD8 T cells will mount an immune response against the cell by releasing chemicals that destroy the entire cell. Because CD8 T cells are programmed to kill cells that display foreign peptides, they are sometimes referred to as killer T cells. This response is the only effective way to prevent the creation of more viruses by the infected cells.

Of course, not all microbes grow in the cytosolic compartment of cells. Some bacteria, such as the *Mycobacteria* that cause tuberculosis, grow in vesicles inside a cell, which are sealed off from the rest of the cell by a membrane. Cells infected in this way tend to be macrophages, which engulf bacteria and naturally form a home for such infections. Bacteria in cell vesicles make proteins that are broken down into peptides within the vesicles. These peptides bind to class II MHC molecules, which then migrate to the vesicles from their origin in the endoplasmic reticulum.

Unlike class I MHC molecules, which must ma-

ture around a peptide, class II molecules remain primed for action once they are synthesized. Peter Cresswell, now at Yale, showed that a special chain of amino acids in the endoplasmic reticulum holds the binding ability of class II MHC molecules in check until the molecules move to the vesicles. This extra chain then falls away, enabling the class II MHC molecules to grab hold of any peptides they find.

The class II MHC molecule then delivers the peptide to the surface of the cell. There the peptide can be recognized by T cells that have the CD4 protein on their surface. Unlike CD8 T cells, CD4 T cells do not directly kill the cell. Rather they activate the cells that have displayed the peptide. For instance, one kind of CD4 T cell, called inflammatory T cells (or Th1), can stimulate a macrophage to kill the *Mycobacteria* inside its own vesicles. It is the loss of this class of CD4 T cells that makes patients who have AIDS so susceptible to diseases such as tuberculosis.

Another kind of CD4 T cell—helper T cells (or Th2)—guides the activity of B cells. When a protein binds to the B cell's receptor, the protein is taken to a vesicle, where it is cleaved into peptides that bind to class II MHC molecules. These complexes are then delivered to the cell surface, so that they can be recognized by the helper T cells. The helper T cells tell the B cell to start making antibody, turning on only those B cells that have bound to antigen. Thus, even antibody production is ultimately controlled by MHC molecules and T cells.

Delivering Peptides to the Cell Surface

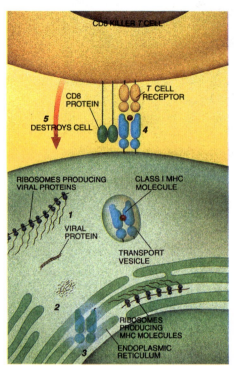

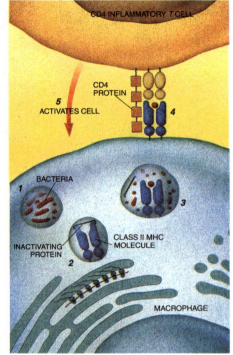

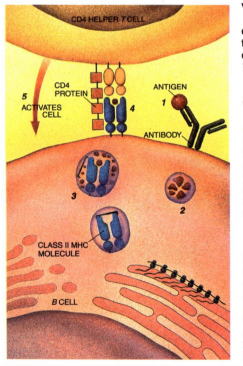

Viral proteins (top left) produced by an infected cell (*1*) are broken down into peptides (*2*). The peptides are taken to the endoplasmic reticulum, where class I MHC molecules form around them (*3*). Each complex goes to the cell surface. There it can be detected by a killer *T* cell, which expresses a CD8 protein (*4*). The *T* cell then secretes compounds that destroy the infected cell (*5*).

The bacteria that infected a macrophage (top right) reside in the cell's vesicle (*1*). A class II MHC molecule, produced in the endoplasmic reticulum, is transported to the vesicle (*2*). A protein chain (*black line*) keeps the molecule inactive until it reaches the vesicle. In the vesicle the chain falls away, enabling the class II MHC molecule to bind to any peptides there (*3*). The complex then moves to the cell surface, where a so-called inflammatory CD4 *T* cell binds to the peptide (*4*). The *T* cell then activates the macrophage, signaling it to destroy the material in its vesicle (*5*).

An antibody on the surface of a *B* cell (left) serves as the *B* cell's receptor. If the antibody discovers a foreign antigen in the bloodstream, it binds to it (*1*) and delivers the antigen to a vesicle inside the cell. The antigen is broken down into peptides (*2*). A class II MHC molecule, which is produced in the endoplasmic reticulum, migrates to the vesicle, where it grabs a peptide (*3*). The MHC molecule transports the peptide to the cell surface (*4*). A CD4 helper *T* cell binds to the antigen and makes molecules that tell the *B* cell to proliferate and to produce antibodies (*5*).

The genes that encode MHC molecules are the most variable ones in humans. This unusual feature of the MHC molecule system may have allowed *Homo sapiens* to survive so many pathogens. Unlike antigen receptor genes, which vary from cell to cell in one person, MHC genes are the same in all of an individual's cells but differ from person to person. Each variant of an MHC molecule will bind different peptides, because the genetic alterations affect mainly the structure of the groove that holds the peptide.

The genetic variability of MHC molecules means that at least some individuals will have MHC molecules that bind to the peptides of any pathogen, even as the structure of microbial proteins evolves. Indeed, A. V. Hill of the University of Oxford has recently studied a population exposed over many hundreds of years to *Plasmodium falciparum*, the parasite that causes fatal malaria. He found that the percentage of people whose MHC molecules bind particularly strongly to peptides from the parasite increased over time. *T* cells can also recognize these genetic difference in MHC molecules, which explains why tissue grafts are rejected: *T* cells in the host regard the peptides bound by a different MHC molecule as foreign and so kill the grafted tissue.

The binding of antigen to receptor is actually only the beginning of the immune response. For a *B* cell to produce antibodies, or a *T* cell to release its killer or helper molecules, the nucleus of the cell must know that binding has occurred at the cell surface. Lymphocyte receptors are made of several proteins that interact to deliver a biochemical message to the cell's interior. When a receptor binds to an antigen, it causes other proteins in the cell membrane to turn on enzymes inside the cell referred to as kinases. Active kinases add compounds called phosphate groups to other proteins inside the cell. The added phosphate groups change the activity of these proteins so that they ultimately signal the cell to grow and differentiate. The CD4 and CD8 proteins on *T* cells, as well as a protein on *B* cells known as CD19, are examples of membrane proteins coupled to kinases inside cells. Another kind of molecule that goes into action is CD45, an enzyme that helps to mediate lymphocyte activation by removing phosphates from certain proteins, thereby deactivating them.

But kinase-mediated signals cannot by themselves activate lymphocytes. Lymphocytes must receive a second signal derived from other cells in the body to grow. These messages are often called costimulatory signals. *B* cells require helper *T* cells not only to recognize antigen but also to make a protein—CD40 ligand—that binds to the B cell molecule CD40. *T* cells rely mainly on so-called B7 molecules as costimulatory signals; such molecules are expressed by the same cells that present antigen (see Figure 3.5). While working in my laboratory, Yang Liu, now at New York University Medical Center, showed that B7 is expressed when the innate immune system recognizes that microbes are present, that is, usually during the early phases of infection. In effect, the innate system may prime the adaptive system for action. In this way, costimulatory signals may also assist the adaptive immune response in differentiating infectious microbes from self-tissues. Lymphocytes that bind to antigen but do not receive costimulation are not activated. As a result, self-antigens alone would not be able to initiate an immune response.

Once a lymphocyte binds to antigen and receives costimulation, it differentiates and becomes active. (The active versions of lymphocytes are sometimes called effector cells, as they actually mediate the immune response.) Once activated, the cell no longer requires the costimulatory signal. Thus, although only cells that express costimulators can elicit an immune response, any cell or molecule can be targeted. This response is important because it enables *B* and *T* cells to attack any cell that has become infected, regardless of its type.

So what is wrong in patients who have agammaglobulinemia, a condition in which antibodies are not made? The answer has only recently been discovered (see Chapter 2, "How the Immune System Develops," by Irving L. Weissman and Max D. Cooper). It turns out that during the development of *B* cells in healthy individuals, the rearrangement of receptor genes is carefully regulated. In other words, the antibody receptor must be manufactured accurately. The V gene for each chain has to be rearranged in the right sequence, and the receptor cannot be completed until all the rearrangements are correctly made.

Thus, to form correct receptors, the cell must determine the state of its receptor genes as development proceeds. A heavy-chain V gene is rearranged so that a cell can make the heavy chain of

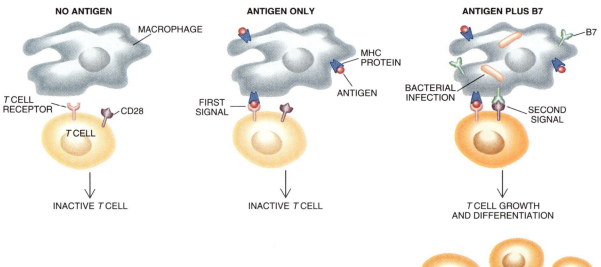

Figure 3.5 STIMULATION by two molecules is needed to activate lymphocytes. The diagrams depict a CD8 *T* cell and a macrophage. Without the presence of antigens, the *T* cell is dormant (*left*). Yet antigen alone cannot induce *T* cell function (*center*). In this way, a response to the body's own antigen does not occur; in fact, this first signal turns off the *T* cell. If the macrophage is infected, it will produce a molecule called B7, which acts on the *T* cell's CD28 surface protein (*right*). Only when an antigen and the B7 molecule are present on the same cell does the *T* cell proliferate.

its receptor first. This chain goes to the cell surface. The presence of the heavy chain at the cell surface signals the *B* cell to stop rearranging heavy-chain genes and to start rearranging light-chain genes. A kinase seems to deliver this crucial message from the cell surface to the interior.

In agammaglobulinemia, heavy chains are made, but light chains are not. In these patients, a kinase has recently been found to be defective. (Interestingly, absence of a related kinase found in *T* cells has an identical effect on *T* cell development.) Apparently, the gene defect described by my father 36 years ago has finally been identified, and we should soon understand how it works.

Meanwhile the kinds of infection that occur in people with agammaglobulinemia have taught us why antibody production is necessary for health. Treatment of these patients with immunoglobulins pooled from donors provides them with antibodies and allows a nearly normal life. But this therapy is only a temporary repair for a genetic disease that can now, in theory, be corrected by inserting the normal gene into a patient's bone marrow cells. Continued strong support for basic research in immunology, genetics, cell biology, cancer and molecular biology is needed to conquer this and the other more prevalent diseases discussed in this book.

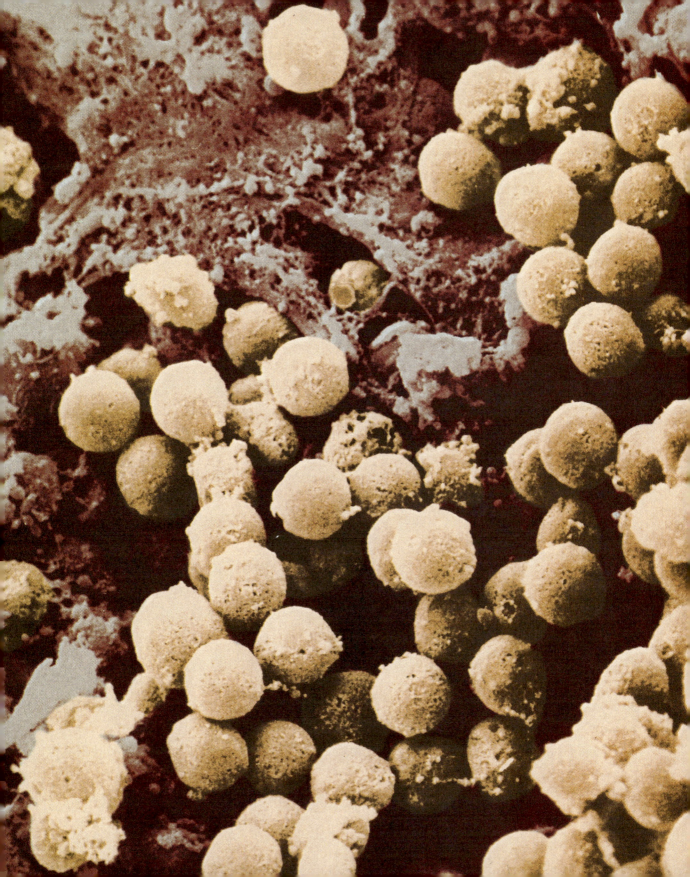

How the Immune System Recognizes the Body

*The human immune system has developed several elegant processes that allow
it to repel foreign invaders and yet not attack the body itself.*

. . .

Philippa Marrack and John W. Kappler

Organisms have various mechanisms of distinguishing between themselves and everything else. Many plants, for example, have hard outer shells that not only protect them against invaders but also define the plants' outer limits. Yeasts have mating-type genes that code for proteins that prevent mating between similar cells. Sponges have a collection of genes whose products can be used to detect and repel alien colonies.

The human body has evolved one of the most elaborate mechanisms for distinguishing invaders from itself. The cells of the immune system—the lymphocytes, macrophages and others—must learn to tolerate every tissue, every cell, every protein in the body. They must be able to distinguish the hemoglobin found in blood from the insulin secreted by the pancreas from the vitreous humor contained in the eye from everything else. They must manage to repel innumerable different kinds of invading organisms and yet not attack the body.

Immunologists have always been preoccupied with the issue of how the body learns to tolerate

itself, but only during the past decade or so have they discovered the details of what prevents the all-important lymphocytes—the *T* cells and the *B* cells—from attacking their host. Many immature lymphocytes have the potential to respond to self-products and therefore pose a threat. The body tries to rid itself of all such cells by resorting to several ingenious processes. If an immune cell reacts to a self-product while it is developing in the thymus or bone marrow, it is usually killed or inactivated (see Figure 4.1). A mature lymphocyte will usually suffer the same fate if it responds to a self-product and does not receive a second chemical message. These basic strategies that the body uses to eliminate self-reacting cells have many variations because there are many different types of lymphocytes and many different kinds of self-products.

Despite the safeguards of the immune system, some self-reacting lymphocytes are not inactivated or killed, and they can cause one of several illnesses known as autoimmune diseases. Immunologists are well aware that if they understood all the mechanisms for tolerance, they might be able to prevent autoimmune diseases. Furthermore, such insights might help surgeons in their continual search for reagents that can prevent the

Figure 4.1 *T* CELLS develop in the thymus, but if one reacts to a protein made by its host before it matures, it will die. The process eliminates many *T* cells that have the potential to attack the body.

immune system from rejecting such transplanted tissues as kidneys, hearts and lungs.

Higher vertebrates have many ways of detecting and destroying invaders. Some of these are relatively nonspecific and depend on the fact that groups of infectious organisms make chemicals that are not produced in large amounts by higher vertebrates. For example, mammals can detect the presence of invading bacteria because bacteria produce peptides that begin with an unusual amino acid—formyl methionine—whereas mammals produce only small amounts of such peptides. Indeed, in mammals, high concentrations of peptides with formyl methionine attract white blood cells called neutrophils, which then consume the bacteria producing the peptides. Similarly, mammals can detect some viruses because viruses produce much greater quantities of double-strand RNA than mammals do. Large amounts of double-strand RNA provoke mammalian cells to produce proteins called interferons, which in turn stimulate a series of reactions that help the host resist further viral infection.

Although these nonspecific responses to chemicals made by bacteria and viruses are an absolutely crucial part of the immune system, vertebrates also require mechanisms for identifying specific invaders. The immune system must be able to recognize foreign products whose chemistry is only slightly different from its own molecules.

The immune system has evolved three very sophisticated methods of recognizing foreign chemicals, or what are termed antigens. The basis of these mechanisms is the three kinds of so-called receptor proteins found on lymphocytes. The first method requires B cells that have receptor proteins known as immunoglobulins; the second relies on T cells that have a receptor protein called alpha-beta, and the third utilizes T cells that have the protein gamma-delta.

Many receptors are attached to the surface of each lymphocyte, and they will, in specific circumstances, bind to antigens. Each receptor is made up of two different polypeptide chains; immunoglobulins consist of so-called light and heavy chains; the alpha-beta protein is made of an alpha chain and a beta chain, whereas the gamma-delta protein has, as you might guess, a gamma chain and a delta chain. Each chain can vary in sequence from one cell to another. For example, the alpha and beta chains of any given T cell will almost certainly differ from those of any other T cell. The receptors of any given T cell, therefore, will probably bind to a different set of materials than those of other T cells. Human beings have as many as a million million T cells and consequently have many different alpha-beta molecules available to recognize foreign material.

Indeed, when one considers the vast number of alpha-beta receptors of T cells as well as the many immunoglobulin molecules of B cells and the many gamma-delta receptors of T cells, it is no small wonder that none of the lymphocytes recognizes products of its own host. This remarkable phenomenon has intrigued investigators for decades, and many theories have been put forward to explain how the human immune system learns to tolerate the cells of the body.

One of the first ideas was that animals simply cannot make lymphocyte receptors that are self-reactive. In particular, humans might not have the genes necessary to create alpha-beta receptors that could react with human proteins. Immunologists have known for many years that this explanation is not right. Nowadays we realize that because the composition and structure of receptors are determined somewhat at random, some receptors are likely to be able to bind to the chemicals of their host.

Randomness is introduced in at least two ways. First, the receptors of lymphocytes are made by random combinations of specialized gene segments. The alpha and beta chains of T cells, for example, are created by a random mixture of gene segments known as V-alpha, J-alpha, V-beta, D-beta and J-beta. Second, short, random segments of DNA are introduced into the assembling genes for the alpha-beta receptor. Thus, the organism has no absolute control over the complete amino acid sequences of the receptors.

Control must be exerted in some other way, at some other stage. One of the first researchers to test this hypothesis was Ray D. Owen of the California Institute of Technology. In 1945 he was studying the inheritance of blood types in cattle. He found that twin cows that shared a placenta were very likely to have the same blood type. This correlation was even seen in one case where the twins had different fathers. Owen concluded that the correlation between blood types was a consequence of the exchange of lymphocytes and other blood cells in utero. Furthermore, he suggested that this early exchange prevented the cows from rejecting each other's blood (see Figure 4.2). Later Sir Peter B. Medawar, Rupert E. Billingham and Leslie Brent of the National Institute for Medical Research in London showed that if blood cells were transferred from an adult mouse into an unrelated, newborn mouse, the newborn could accept a skin graft from the adult later in its life. Hence, the introduction of blood cells at birth could affect the ability of the individual to accept not only blood but also skin.

Most important, this work and Owen's research led to the same broad conclusion: the immune system is not born with all the instructions needed to recognize the products of its host; rather it learns what is self as it develops.

One of the first ideas that explained how the immune system learns tolerance to self was put forward by Joshua Lederberg, now at the Rockefeller University. In 1959 he suggested that immature lymphocytes may not react to antigens in the same way that mature lymphocytes do. Usually if something binds to the immunoglobulin of a mature B cell, the lymphocyte changes into an antibody-secreting cell; if a molecule attaches to the receptors of a mature T cell, the lymphocyte becomes either a cytokine-secreting cell or a killer cell. Lederberg postulated that if an antigen binds to the receptor of an immature cell, the cell might die instead of becoming active (see Figure 4.3).

Lederberg's hypothesis—now called clonal deletion theory—provides a mechanism for eliminating lymphocytes that react to self-products. The process works in the following way. T and B cells are produced constantly throughout the lifetime of the individual, even though the production of T cells may slow down after adolescence. Regardless of when they are produced, T and B cells will always develop surrounded by a sea of materials produced by the host. Those immature cells whose receptors recognize self-products are destroyed, according to the theory; consequently, only lymphocytes that are not self-reactive will develop to maturity (see Figure 4.4). To be sure, the immature lymphocytes will also die if they bind to a foreign antigen, but an immune response will be carried out by those lymphocytes that matured before the infection.

Some time after the clonal deletion theory was proposed, researchers came up with two other plausible explanations for why the immune system is tolerant to its host. One suggestion was that a developing lymphocyte might be inactivated permanently, instead of dying, when its receptors were engaged. (Immunologists describe an inactive lymphocyte as "anergic.") The other hypothesis stated that self-reactive T and B cells might be

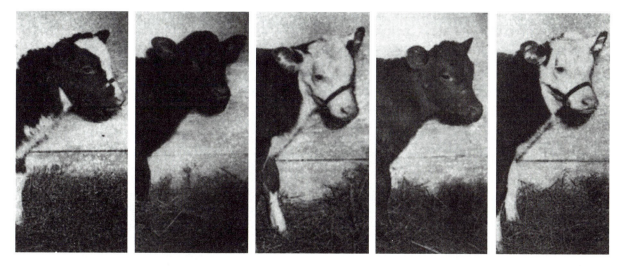

Figure 4.2 QUINTUPLET COWS gave some of the first evidence that the immune system learns to tolerate self-products. The fetal cows shared a single placenta in their mother's womb and exchanged blood. As a result, the calfs accepted blood from one another.

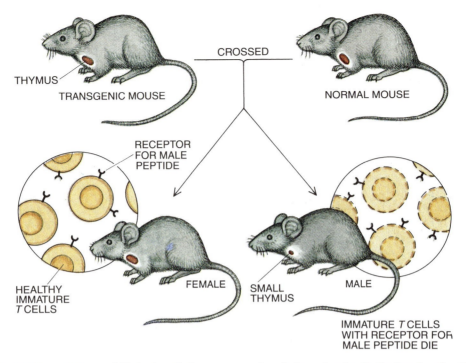

Figure 4.3 IMMATURE *T* CELLS are killed when their receptors bind to peptides, as shown by experiments with genetically engineered mice. The mice were designed to harbor *T* cells whose receptors could recognize a peptide made only in male mice. In the female mice, *T* cells developed normally. In the male mice, *T* cells were absent because the young *T* cells apparently bound to the peptide and died.

kept at bay by lymphocytes called suppressor cells.

For many years, researchers struggled to distinguish among these three hypotheses. Lymphocytes are clearly very good at recognizing foreign tissue. For example, a human being will reject skin grafts from an unrelated person very rapidly, whereas an individual will accept skin tissue transplanted from one part of the body to another. Likewise, in culture dishes, lymphocytes fail to be activated by other cells from their host but react violently to lymphocytes or cells from another individual. Yet the outstanding issue remained: Does the immune system fail to respond to self-products because the potentially reactive lymphocytes are simply not there or are inactive or are being suppressed by other cells?

To resolve this question, workers attempted to devise methods for identifying lymphocytes that recognized particular antigens but did not necessarily respond by dividing. The development of these techniques turned out to be a daunting task.

If the *T* and *B* cells of an animal have never been exposed to a specific antigen, only a small fraction of the lymphocytes should have the potential to react to that antigen. The "frequency" of reacting cells, as immunologists say, is somewhere around one in a million. Indeed, the frequency is so low that it would be impossible to distinguish the few lymphocytes that might recognize self-products from the many that do not.

Nevertheless, researchers have recently developed two experimental tools that circumvent this problem. The first requires a peculiar type of antigen called a superantigen, whereas the second relies on genetically altered animals known as transgenic mice. Both the superantigen techniques and the experiments with transgenic animals deserve to be described in some detail.

Whether a superantigen, or antigen, will bind to a lymphocyte depends ultimately on the composition and structure of the receptor. The alpha-beta receptor, for example, is a somewhat

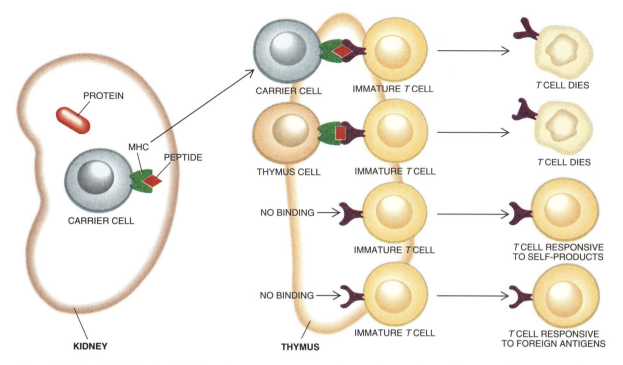

Figure 4.4 DEATH OF YOUNG *T* CELLS that bind to self-proteins helps to prevent the immune system from attacking the body. *T* cells are exposed to most self-products as they develop in the thymus. Some self-proteins are made in the thymus, whereas others are carried there, from organs such as the kidney, by traveling cells. Those young *T* cells whose receptors bind to self-products die. Because some self-products never reach the thymus, some self-reactive cells reach maturity.

random assembly of such segments as V-alpha and V-beta. The receptor is designed mainly to recognize foreign peptides, that is, antigens made by breaking down proteins from invading organisms. The receptor, however, will bind only to a foreign peptide that has already been attached to one of the major histocompatibility complex (MHC) proteins—specialized molecules found on the surface of ordinary cells. As far as researchers can tell, all the variable segments of the alpha-beta receptor play a role in binding the MHC protein and its captured foreign peptide. To recognize a specific antigen, a *T* cell must have a receptor with exactly the right combination of variable segments.

Superantigens are a different story. Like their ordinary counterparts, superantigens will attach to a particular type of MHC molecule, but they will then bind to a specific V-beta segment of an alpha-beta receptor, almost regardless of the structure of the rest of the receptor (see Figure 4.5). Because the number of different types of V-beta segments is small compared with the number of different alpha-beta receptors, many more *T* cells are capable of recognizing a particular superantigen than are able to identify a specific antigen. In mice, for example, the number of different V-beta segments totals about 20, and thus any particular V-beta can be found in about one in every 20 *T* cells that have alpha-beta receptors.

Most important, because so many *T* cells respond to a specific superantigen, researchers can observe the reaction. To do so, they first obtain an antibody that can bind to the V-beta target of a superantigen. The antibody is then tagged with a molecule that fluoresces under ultraviolet light. Hence, the fluorescent antibody will attach to *T* cells that respond to the superantigen, and workers can identify the cells using a microscope or a fluorescent-activated cell sorter.

To test this technique, investigators first used a superantigen produced by the mouse mammary tumor virus. Mice become infected with the virus

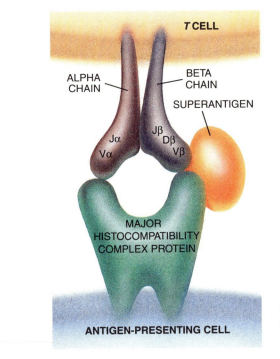

T CELL

ALPHA CHAIN

BETA CHAIN

SUPERANTIGEN

Jα
Vα

Jβ
Dβ
Vβ

MAJOR HISTOCOMPATIBILITY COMPLEX PROTEIN

ANTIGEN-PRESENTING CELL

Figure 4.5 SUPERANTIGEN binds to only one part of a T cell's receptor, in this case the region known as V-beta. Before the superantigen attaches to the receptor, it must bind to a major histocompatibility complex protein on the surface of a cell.

through the milk of their mothers. The virus invades the lymphocytes of mice by manufacturing a superantigen and stimulating the lymphocyte. The mouse mammary tumor virus, like the virus that causes AIDS, is a retrovirus. Such viruses contain genes made of RNA, but they reproduce by making DNA copies of their RNA. This DNA is inserted into the DNA of infected cells. The viral DNA then gives rise to viral RNA and proteins—materials that assemble to form new infectious viruses.

Occasionally, retroviruses infect the cells that produce sperm or eggs. If that happens, the virus may become part of the DNA of the offspring and may cease to be an infectious organism. In fact, nearly all mice have one or more mammary tumor viruses integrated into their DNA. These viral integrants then generate proteins that are, for all intents and purposes, self-products. The viral proteins are made constantly throughout the life span of the animal, just as genuine self-proteins are.

We and our colleagues at the National Jewish Center for Immunology and Respiratory Medicine in Denver used the superantigens produced by these viral integrants to test how the immune system responds to self-products, since, as far as the mouse is concerned, the proteins made by the integrant are self-products. In 1988 we and several other research teams began to examine the effects of the superantigen made by MTV-7, a strain of mammary tumor virus that has naturally integrated into the DNA of some mice. This superantigen reacts with certain V-beta segments on the receptors of mouse T cells. Specifically, the superantigen binds to the segments known as V-beta 6, V-beta 7, V-beta 8.1 and V-beta 9.

Working with Uwe Staerz, then at the Basel Institute for Immunology, we focused on the effects of the MTV-7 superantigen on V-beta 8.1. We found that in mice whose DNA is free of MTV-7, as much as 8 percent of T cells have V-beta 8.1 as part of their receptors. On the other hand, mice whose DNA includes MTV-7 did not harbor any mature T cells with V-beta 8.1. At the same time, a Swiss research team—including H. Robson MacDonald of the Ludwig Institute for Cancer Research in Lausanne and Rolf M. Zinkernagel and Hans Hengartner of the University of Zurich—reported that T cells bearing V-beta 6 are also missing in mice whose DNA has MTV-7. More recently

Edward Palmer and his colleagues at the National Jewish Center obtained similar results for V-beta 9, and we discovered the same for V-beta 7.

All these experiments showed that the superantigen made by integrated MTV-7 somehow leads to the disappearance of T cells that can react with the superantigen. So, in this case, T cells that can recognize self-products are neither inactivated nor suppressed by other cells; the T cells are simply not there and must have died at some stage in their development.

T cells begin as precursor cells. During the fetal stage of animal development, the precursors originate in the yolk sac or liver, whereas young and adult animals spawn precursors in their bone marrow. These cells migrate to the thymus where they start to build the genes that contain the instructions for making alpha chains, beta chains and other receptor-related proteins. Soon after, as alpha-beta receptors start to appear in small quantities on the surface of the cells, the precursors become immature thymocytes. Such cells then go through a mysterious stage of development referred to as positive selection. In this stage the immature thymocytes add an increasing number of alpha-beta receptors to their surfaces.

As we discovered, however, an immature thymocyte will die in the thymus if it recognizes the superantigen produced by integrated MTV-7. Many different experiments on different animals have now shown that superantigens cause the death of immature thymocytes about halfway through their development.

Although these results offered strong support for the clonal deletion theory, immunologists were forced to entertain the possibility that superantigens, which have so many special properties, do not affect T cells in the same way as normal antigens do. Harald von Boehmer and Michael Steinmetz and their collaborators at the University of Basel and Hoffmann–La Roche therefore approached the problem of self-tolerance in a completely different way. They used transgenic mice, which are produced by the injection of DNA into fertilized mouse eggs. Such DNA is frequently incorporated into the DNA of the developing embryo and is passed on to progeny.

Using this technique, von Boehmer and his colleagues created mice in which most of the T cells had the same alpha-beta receptor. To understand how they accomplished this, one must know that

as a precursor T cell develops in an ordinary mouse, the cell actually builds the DNA that yields a particular alpha-beta receptor. Pieces of the DNA coding for the receptor are contained within the DNA of all mouse cells, but only in developing T cells are the pieces rearranged into functional genes. Von Boehmer isolated DNA that coded for a specific alpha-beta receptor gene, which had already been rearranged. He then injected mouse eggs with the rearranged DNA. As the mice developed, the rearranged DNA took precedence over the unrearranged receptor genes. Hence, most T cells in the transgenic mice bore the receptor created by the injected genes.

The receptor that von Boehmer chose to make was one that would bind an antigen present only in male mice, provided that the antigen was accompanied by the MHC protein D^b. In those mice that made D^b, he and his co-workers found, as expected, an undeniable difference between the females and males. In the female mice, many T cells had the introduced receptor on their surfaces. In the male mice, however, cells bearing the receptor were almost completely missing; they had apparently been destroyed at an early stage of their development in the thymus.

These findings show that Lederberg was right when he proposed the clonal deletion theory. Immature lymphocytes go through a stage when binding of their receptors causes them to die. Self-reactive cells are killed before they have a chance to proliferate and damage their host. The immune system does indeed use clonal deletion to establish tolerance to self.

Unfortunately, the clonal deletion theory does not address the problem of how the immune system learns to tolerate self-products that the thymus either does not make or produces in extremely small quantities. This concern applies not only to proteins that are relatively sequestered, such as those made in the brain or eye, but also to proteins that are made only in certain specialized tissues.

In fact, many of these unusual self-antigens are transported to the thymus. Monocytes and B cells can take up a protein in one part of the body and carry it to another—to the thymus in particular. This kind of process accounts very well for how the immune system learns to tolerate many self-products that are not generated in the thymus.

Yet this scheme does not apply in all cases; for instance, it does not explain how T cells learn to tolerate peptides that bind to class I MHC proteins. Such MHC proteins attach only to peptides that are derived from proteins made within the cell itself. Monocytes and B cells are thus incapable of transporting the peptides of other cells to the thymus. Immature T cells in the thymus are not exposed to some cytoplasmic proteins and so have no way of learning to tolerate them. Some other mechanism must be at work that either kills, inactivates or suppresses mature T cells.

Scientists have searched for a mechanism by which mature T cells could learn tolerance. Several different experiments have now shown that when mature T cells encounter self-products, they may either die or become inactive.

One such experiment was conducted by Jacques F.A.P. Miller and his colleagues at the Walter and Eliza Hall Institute of Medical Research in Australia. They worked with a gene for a class I MHC protein known as K^b. They introduced this gene into a mouse in such a way that the gene was controlled by the insulin gene. Hence, the mouse made K^b only in its cells that normally make insulin, that is, the beta cells of the pancreas. Because these cells are immobile, K^b could not find its way to the thymus of these animals, and, not surprisingly, the thymocytes of these mice could bind to K^b. Mature T cells could not respond, however, unless they were confronted with K^b under very special circumstances. These results showed that sometimes mature T cells that can recognize self-antigens can survive in animals but become anergic. Furthermore, in other experiments Susan Webb and her collaborators at the Scripps Research Institute in La Jolla, Calif., have shown that under some conditions, mature T cells die when exposed to self-antigen.

Immunologists do not know exactly what causes death rather than inactivation of mature T cells. Perhaps the inactive cells are just intermediates on their way to the grave. In any case, the important outcome is that these cells cannot respond. Indeed, researchers have now gathered so many examples of antigens' causing the death or inactivation of T cells that they are quite puzzled about why and when antigens from invading organisms cause T cells to become active. T cells with alpha-beta receptors seem to have been designed so that they will not usually be activated when their receptors are engaged. The question is, therefore, how a mature T cell decides whether to divide, become

inactive or die when its receptors react to something.

The issue was resolved in part by a classic experiment performed some 30 years ago by David W. Dresser, then at the Medical Research Council Laboratories in England. At the time, investigators were well aware that the immune system responds vigorously to aggregated preparations of foreign protein or to protein mixed with an adjuvant, such as dead bacteria in mineral oil. Dresser found, however, that the immune system fails to respond to soluble foreign proteins. In fact, once the immune system is exposed to a soluble foreign protein, it will subsequently fail to react to any preparation of that protein. The system learns to tolerate soluble foreign proteins, at least in part, because it eliminates the T cells that can respond to such proteins, as was discovered in 1971 by Jacques M. Chiller and William O. Weigle of the Scripps Clinic and Roger Taylor of the MRC Laboratories.

Evidently, T cells can recognize the form of the antigen, although how they do so was not clear until recently. Alpha-beta receptors do not have a direct way of detecting in what form the foreign protein was introduced into the body. As long as a peptide is attached to an MHC protein, it can bind to an alpha-beta receptor regardless of whether the peptide came from a protein in solution or in an adjuvant. Something besides the alpha-beta receptor must be giving the T cell information about the form of the antigen.

In 1970 Peter A. Bretscher and Melvin Cohn of the Salk Institute for Biological Studies suggested a solution to the problem in an early form, and five years later Kevin J. Lafferty and Alistair J. Cunningham of the John Curtin School of Medical Research in Australia reformulated the idea into its currently accepted form. In immunologic terms, T cells need two signals to be stimulated by an antigen: the first signal comes from the binding of the alpha-beta receptor, and the second is from something else (see Figure 4.6).

The task of identifying this second signal has preoccupied immunologists for the past decade. One clue came from the work of Ronald H. Schwartz and his collaborators at the National Institutes of Health [see "T Cell Anergy," by Ronald H. Schwartz; SCIENTIFIC AMERICAN, August 1993]. In 1987 his group demonstrated that antigens bound to MHC proteins will not provoke cultured T cells to divide if the cells that bear those MHC proteins are prepared in a certain way. Not only

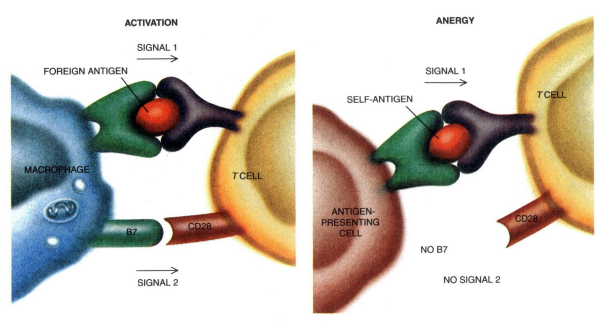

ACTIVATION

SIGNAL 1

FOREIGN ANTIGEN

MACROPHAGE

T CELL

B7   CD28

SIGNAL 2

ANERGY

SIGNAL 1

T CELL

SELF-ANTIGEN

ANTIGEN-
PRESENTING
CELL

CD28

NO B7

NO SIGNAL 2

Figure 4.6 IMMUNE SYSTEM has a safety mechanism that prevents a mature *T* cell from mounting an immune attack against its host. Before a *T* cell can attack, it must receive two signals. The first is the binding of an antigen to the *T* cell's receptor. The second is typically the secretion and binding of a protein, B7, for example (*left*). If a *T* cell is exposed to a self-protein that is presented on a nonstimulatory cell, the *T* cell will die or become inactive (*right*).

did the *T* cells fail to respond, but they were also unable to divide several days later when confronted with antigens bound to MHC proteins on live, unprepared cells. The prepared cells bearing the MHC proteins had somehow inactivated the *T* cells.

Later work has shown that the mechanism of inactivation involves CD28, a protein on the surface of *T* cells. When CD28 binds to a protein known as B7 or BB1—which resides on the surface of *B* cells and macrophages—it delivers a signal to the *T* cell. Normally, a *T* cell binds an antigen and an MHC protein and a B7 at the same time. Consequently, the *T* cell gets two signals: one through its receptor and another through CD28. If a *T* cell is confronted with an antigen on a cell that does not have functional B7, it will get the receptor signal without the CD28 signal. The *T* cell is thereby inactivated. This finding lends strong support for the theory that *T* cells require two signals to respond to an antigen. (It is worth emphasizing, however, that CD28-B7 is only one of many possible secondary signals.)

Of course, the way the CD28-B7 signal is blocked in the laboratory is not the way it happens in the immune system. Researchers are still figuring out what cells can present antigens on MHC proteins but fail to deliver the C28-B7 signal. The answer may be *B* cells, as suggested by such investigators as David C. Parker of the University of Massachusetts at Worcester and Polly C. Matzinger of the National Institute of Allergy and Infectious Diseases. Most *B* cells in animals bear very little, if any, B7. Only after the *B* cells have been stimulated themselves do they increase their production of B7 to measurable amounts. Therefore, if *T* cells encounter antigen on *B* cells, they may be inactivated because they receive one signal without another. At the present, this theory seems plausible, but it has not been proved. Most likely, only certain specialized cells—macrophages, dendritic cells and perhaps activated *B* cells—can deliver both the first and second signals to *T* cells, thereby activating them.

The body has many ways to deal with a self-reactive *T* cell that has an alpha-beta receptor. If the cell is still developing in the thymus and its receptor binds to a self-product, it will die. On the other hand, a mature cell whose receptor binds to a self-product will be inactivated or killed if it fails to receive a second message, such as the CD28-B7 signal. Investigators are less certain about how *B* cells and *T* cells with gamma-delta receptors respond to self-products.

The immune system seems to handle self-reactive *B* cells and their immunoglobulin proteins in much the same way as it takes care of self-reactive *T* cells with alpha-beta receptors. For example, in 1976 Norman R. Klinman and his colleagues at the University of Pennsylvania and Ellen Vitetta and her co-workers at the University of Texas Southwestern Medical Center at Dallas independently showed that immature *B* cells in tissue culture could be made tolerant to antigen much more easily than mature *B* cells could. Later, Sir Gustav J. V. Nossal and his collaborators at the Hall Institute showed that this phenomenon could involve *B* cell anergy as well as *B* cell death.

Recently researchers have been able to demonstrate this phenomenon in animals rather than in tissue culture dishes, using transgenic mice. For the experiments, they injected fertilized mouse eggs with fully rearranged, mature genes for a particular immunoglobulin, thereby introducing the genes into the mouse DNA. As *B* cells matured in the developing mice, the introduced genes caused almost all the *B* cells to produce the specific immunoglobulin on their surface.

Among the first researchers to try this technique were Christopher C. Goodnow and his colleagues at the University of Sydney. The workers created two groups of transgenic animals. One contained the genes for an immunoglobulin that binds to the foreign protein hen egg lysozyme. The other group contained a gene that instructs cells to produce hen egg lysozyme. When mice from one group were allowed to mate with mice from the other group, they produced offspring whose DNA contained both types of gene. Hence, the offspring had the ability to make both hen egg lysozyme and the immunoglobulin that binds to hen egg lysozyme. The investigators found that *B* cells in the offspring were inactivated, confirming the results found in tissue culture dishes (see Figure 4.7).

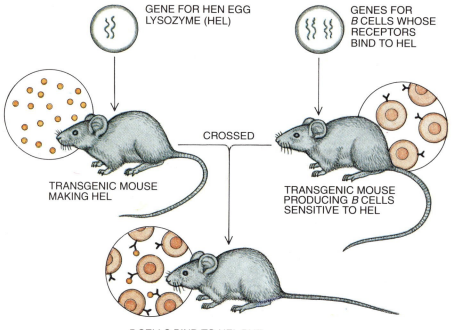

GENE FOR HEN EGG LYSOZYME (HEL)

GENES FOR *B* CELLS WHOSE RECEPTORS BIND TO HEL

CROSSED

TRANSGENIC MOUSE MAKING HEL

TRANSGENIC MOUSE PRODUCING *B* CELLS SENSITIVE TO HEL

B CELLS BIND TO HEL BUT DO NOT BECOME ACTIVE

Figure 4.7 YOUNG *B* CELLS become inactive when they bind to something, as shown by experiments with transgenic mice. A group of mice was engineered to produce a protein found in chicken: hen egg lysozyme (HEL). Other mice were designed to make *B* cells with receptors that bind to HEL. The two groups of mice were mated, producing mice that produced HEL and *B* cells sensitive to HEL. *B* cells in these animals could not be activated by reagents that usually stimulate such cells.

A similar experiment was performed by David Nemazee, then at the Basel Institute for Immunology, and Kurt Buerki of Sandoz Pharma. They made transgenic mice with a gene for an immunoglobulin molecule that binds to the MHC protein D^b. Some of the transgenic mice naturally produce D^b in their bone marrow. In those mice, the B cells died.

Why are the immature B cells sometimes inactivated and sometimes killed by contact with self-antigen? Investigators have found that the form of the antigen determines the fate of the cells. Soluble antigens, such as hen egg lysozyme, are more likely to inactivate immature B cells that bind to them. On the other hand, cell-bound aggregated antigens, such as D^b, are more likely to kill immature B cells.

All in all, tolerance mechanisms for B cells are very similar to those for alpha-beta T cells. Immature B cells die or are inactivated when their receptors bind to something. Whether tolerance can also be imposed on mature B cells, as it can on mature T cells, remains to be determined.

In contrast to B cells, T cells that have gamma-delta receptors are a mystery. In humans and mice, there are about as many of these cells as B cells or alpha-beta T cells, and the gamma-delta T cells are clearly very important. Yet scientists have only an incomplete picture of how these cells contribute to the immune system. Gamma-delta T cells seem to respond to products that are made by the host when, for example, tissue is abraded, overheated, exposed to dangerous metals or attacked by invading organisms. The receptors on these cells appear to have been designed particularly to bind to certain components of self. If this is true, investigators are then faced with the problem of how these self-reactive cells are kept under control. At the moment, they have no idea.

A healthy immune system does not attack its own host. Unfortunately, the immune system makes mistakes, and T cells and B cells that can respond to self-antigens sometimes appear. These cells damage the body they occupy, leading to such diseases as rheumatoid arthritis, multiple sclerosis and lupus. At the moment, physicians treat these diseases by waging a full-scale battle against the immune cells that cause them. Powerful anti-inflammatory drugs and chemicals that kill or slow down activated T and B cells are used to keep the autoimmune response in check. Sadly, these methods are not always effective and in some cases have unwanted side effects. Immunologists hope that if they continue to study how the immune system learns to tolerate the body, they will find ways to improve the treatment of autoimmune diseases.

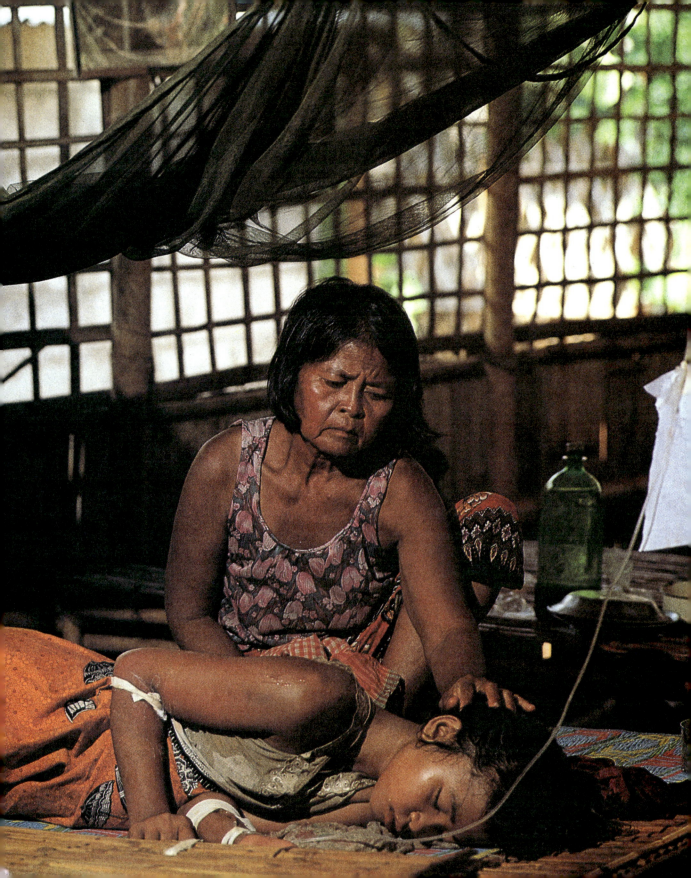

Infectious Diseases and the Immune System

When bacteria, viruses and other pathogens infect the body, they hide in different places.
Each component of the immune system is most adept at rousting trespassers from one location.

• • •

William E. Paul

Throughout the world infectious diseases have always been the leading cause of human death. Malaria, tuberculosis, infectious diarrhea and many other illnesses still exact an awful toll in suffering and mortality, particularly in the developing world. For a time, it was widely assumed that infectious diseases had been brought under control in at least the industrialized nations. Yet the appearance of AIDS and the recent resurgence of tuberculosis, including the evolution of strains resistant to many drugs, vividly illustrate that the monster was not slain but merely asleep (see Figure 5.1).

Notwithstanding those grim truths, the power of the immune system to deal with infection is remarkable—particularly when enhanced by modern vaccine technology. Because of a concerted global vaccination effort, smallpox has been completely eradicated: the last case from a natural infection occurred in Somalia in 1977. There is hope for a similar success in the control of polio. The

World Health Organization has set a goal of eradicating polio by the year 2000; the disease may have already been eliminated from the Western Hemisphere. Those triumphs underscore the need to use the vaccines we now possess to their full effectiveness and to develop vaccines against those diseases that still remain great public health problems.

Perhaps the key to further success lies in a keener appreciation of how the immune system responds to infectious agents. The highly sophisticated immunologic defenses seen in humans and other higher organisms were shaped through evolution by the perpetual struggle between diverse, extremely mutable microorganisms and their hosts. The struggle is reenacted within each individual: a person's immune armament meets innumerable challenges in a lifetime, foiling countless opponents, and a fatal infection often represents the only unqualified loss in a generally victorious campaign.

An individual's immune response can be tailored to the challenges that person encounters because its mechanisms, like its foes, are diverse and specific. Lymphocytes can detect invading organisms because they are equipped with surface receptor molecules; the genes for those receptors can be shuffled and varied to produce structures that match virtually any foreign substance. In addition, the varied cells that make up the immune

Figure 5.1 MALARIA and other infectious diseases continue to be major scourges, particularly in developing nations. Here a woman at the border between Thailand and Cambodia cares for a girl suffering from cerebral malaria. When bacteria, parasites and viruses colonize different environments inside the body, they rely on a variety of tricks to evade the immune system. The immune system, in turn, has developed countermeasures.

system specialize in their functions. These specializations endow vertebrates with the capacity to recognize and eliminate (or at least control) microorganisms that establish themselves in different microenvironments within the body. The complexity of the immune response—the very feature that gives it extraordinary flexibility and clout—poses daunting challenges to those who would decipher it.

With that in mind, it is instructive to describe the current understanding of the immune response in relation to various types of infection. In a broad sense, each of the immune system's components appears to be directed against agents that infect one niche in the human body. The immunologic proteins called antibodies, for example, are especially effective at destroying bacteria that live outside human cells—in, say, the blood or the fluid surrounding lung cells. The white blood cells known as CD4 *T* lymphocytes are of central importance in defeating the bacteria and other parasites that live within cells, especially those found in the organelles that are their pathway of entry into the cells. Another class of white blood cells, the CD8 *T* lymphocytes, routs pathogens such as viruses that associate even more intimately with the cellular machinery of the host.

Of course, this view of the immune system is a vast oversimplification; the most protective immune responses involve all the system's components acting in concert. In practice, each part may be involved, directly or indirectly, in repelling almost any type of infection. The CD4 *T* cells, for example, are often loosely called helper *T* cells because they secrete substances that amplify and control virtually all aspects of immunity. Nevertheless, this simplified scheme does afford insights into the principal responses in the battle against pathogens.

A look at the infection that causes pneumococcal pneumonia highlights the protective importance of antibodies. When the bacterium *Streptococcus pneumoniae* (also referred to as the pneumococcus) enters the lungs, it colonizes the space in the alveoli, the microscopic sacs where oxygen is transferred into the blood and carbon dioxide is removed (see Figure 5.2). The pneumococcus multiplies there, causing tissue damage and inflammation that can impair breathing. If the bacterial infection goes unchecked, complications can develop, and in a substantial fraction of cases the patient will die.

Because they live outside of cells and very near the bloodstream, pneumococci would seem to be

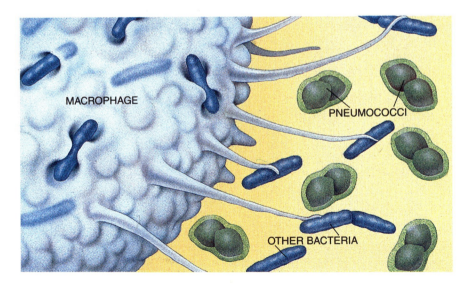

Figure 5.2 PNEUMOCOCCI are bacteria that can cause potentially fatal infections by colonizing spaces inside the lungs. Without assistance from antibodies and complement proteins, macrophages cannot destroy pneumococci, be- **cause complex sugar molecules in the capsules surrounding the bacteria prevent the macrophages from adhering to them.**

easy prey for the macrophages, neutrophils and other phagocytic cells of the immune system that scavenge the body for bacteria and debris. Instead the pneumococcal bacteria escape detection because they are surrounded by capsules of complex sugar molecules, or polysaccharides. Phagocytes cannot bind to these polysaccharides and consequently cannot ingest *S. pneumoniae.*

The capsular polysaccharides offer a much more attractive target, however, for the antibody-producing white blood cells called *B* lymphocytes. The surface membranes of *B* cells bristle with receptors for certain determinants of foreign substances, or antigens. Each *B* cell carries receptors for only one kind of antigenic determinant. But because the body produces billions of *B* cells, most with receptors of distinct structure and specificity, the chances are good that at least some *B* cells will bear receptors that can bind to the antigens presented by a microbial invader.

Invariably, then, some *B* cells have receptors for antigenic determinants of the polysaccharide capsule of *S. pneumoniae* (see boxed figure "How the Immune System Attacks Pneumococci"). Because the molecular structures of the polysaccharides are repetitive, the same capsule antigens appear frequently. Consequently, many receptors on a single *B* cell will latch onto the capsule simultaneously, which brings them into proximity on the cell surface. Such receptor aggregation is essential for the activation of the *B* cells in response to polysaccharide antigens, and it elicits a potent *B* cell response.

Once a *B* cell has been activated in this way, rapid biochemical events occur within it. Enzymes called tyrosine kinases catalyze changes in intracellular signal molecules, such as some proteins associated with the receptors. Ultimately, this cascade of reactions prompts the *B* cells to divide and to secrete antibodies against the capsule polysaccharides. (Certain chemical signals, or cytokines, supplied by helper *T* cells also seem to be essential to the full mobilization of the *B* cell defense.)

The antibodies released by an activated *B* cell bind to the capsule around the pneumococci and improve the ability of phagocytes to ingest them. The precise means by which this result is achieved depends on the structural and chemical characteristics of the antibody molecules. Antibodies belonging to the immunoglobulin G (IgG) class of proteins have a region designated Fc-gamma. Macrophages and other phagocytes have receptor molecules that bind specifically to the Fc-gamma region and that, when engaged, signal the macrophage to ingest the attached particle. These antibodies thus give the phagocytes the "handholds" they need to attack the pneumococci and end the infection.

Polysaccharide-bound antibodies can also make the pneumococci more vulnerable by activating a cascade of circulating enzymes referred to as the complement system. Fragments of one of the enzymes, known as C3, can bind firmly to the bacterial surface. Receptors on the phagocytes can then recognize the C3 fragments—much as the Fc-gamma receptors bind to IgG antibodies—and augment their action against the pneumococci. Because the binding of even one antibody to the pneumococcal capsule can set off complement reactions, antibodies act as a powerful amplifying signal for inducing phagocytosis. Furthermore, researchers have recently shown that the presence of complement fragments on an antigen also markedly increases the efficiency with which *B* cells will be stimulated by that antigen, which means that the complement system also increases the production of antibodies. Because of the positive feedback inherent in this arrangement, the line of defense offered by antibodies is extraordinarily rapid and effective.

The antibody response is in many respects the simplest in the immune system's repertoire. It is a straightforward race between antibody production and pathogen replication, a case of "the quick or the dead." The response is well suited to fighting pneumococcal pneumonia and other infections caused by extracellular bacteria; *B* cells and antibodies specialize in nabbing conspicuous invaders. The resistance to infection that develops in people who have been vaccinated or previously exposed to an infectious agent also depends primarily on the antibody response.

Many microbes, however, establish infections inside cells, where antibodies and complement cannot reach them. Antibodies may have a chance to control such an invader while it is en route to its intracellular destination, but that response may not be prompt or vigorous enough to prevent the pathogen from gaining entry to cells—especially if the host has never before been exposed to the pathogen. The situation calls for different protective strategies, ones that can recognize a covert attack.

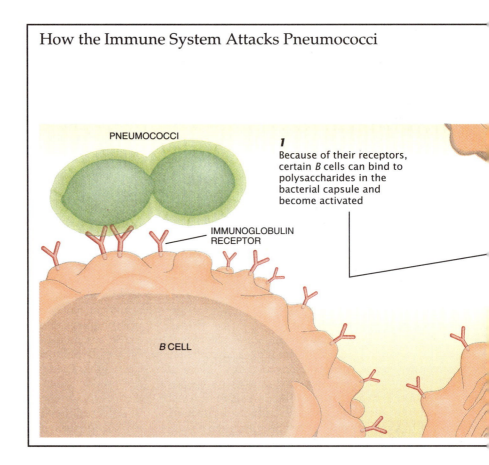

How the Immune System Attacks Pneumococci

PNEUMOCOCCI

IMMUNOGLOBULIN
RECEPTOR

B CELL

1
Because of their receptors, certain *B* cells can bind to polysaccharides in the bacterial capsule and become activated

Such intracellular infections can be thought of as taking two forms. In one, the infectious microorganisms are found within the membrane-bound organelles (endosomes and lysosomes) through which they entered the cell. This behavior is typical of the bacteria that cause tuberculosis and leprosy. In the other form of infection, the microorganism gains access to the fluid part of the cell (the cytosol) and the cell nucleus. Viruses are the most common of these intracellular pathogens. The *T* cells provide the main defense against both types of infections, although the means by which they control or eradicate each one are quite different.

Perhaps the simplest and clearest illustration of how *T* cells fight intracellular infections can be drawn from studies involving the parasitic protozoa *Leishmania*. The principal diseases caused by *Leishmania*, visceral and cutaneous leishmaniasis, may be less well known to Western readers than is tuberculosis, but they are common ailments in much of the developing world. Patients who have

visceral leishmaniasis, or kala-azar, as it is often called, suffer from enlarged spleens and livers and low white blood cell counts; they lose their appetites and begin to waste away. Left untreated, the disease can be fatal. Cutaneous leishmaniasis is marked by ulcerated skin lesions that generally heal but that may take a year or more to do so. In some cases, the lesions may spread to the mucous membranes of the nose and throat, with disfiguring consequences.

The primary target of the *Leishmania* parasite is the macrophage. During their routine scavenging in the bloodstream, macrophages engulf *Leishmania* organisms and package them in vacuoles. Those vacuoles fuse with others that contain proteolytic (protein-splitting) enzymes that can kill and digest most microbes. *Leishmania*, however, differentiate into a new form that not only can endure this chemical assault but actually can thrive during it. The parasites multiply inside the vacuole until the infected macrophage host can no longer sustain them all and dies (see Figure 5.3).

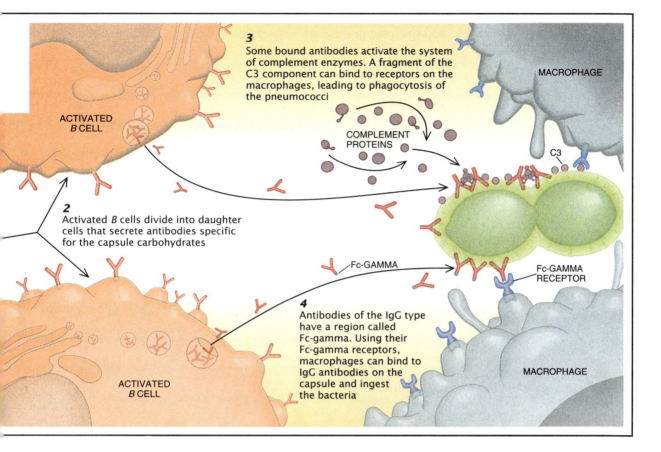

3
Some bound antibodies activate the system of complement enzymes. A fragment of the C3 component can bind to receptors on the macrophages, leading to phagocytosis of the pneumococci

MACROPHAGE

ACTIVATED B CELL

COMPLEMENT PROTEINS

C3

2
Activated B cells divide into daughter cells that secrete antibodies specific for the capsule carbohydrates

Fc-GAMMA

Fc-GAMMA RECEPTOR

4
Antibodies of the IgG type have a region called Fc-gamma. Using their Fc-gamma receptors, macrophages can bind to IgG antibodies on the capsule and ingest the bacteria

ACTIVATED B CELL

MACROPHAGE

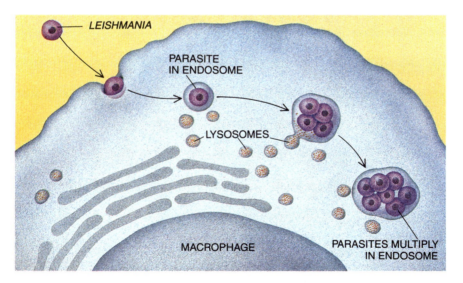

LEISHMANIA

PARASITE IN ENDOSOME

LYSOSOMES

PARASITES MULTIPLY IN ENDOSOME

MACROPHAGE

Figure 5.3 *LEISHMANIA* and many other parasites proliferate inside the organelles of cells, where they are beyond the reach of antibodies. Macrophages ingest *Leishmania* organisms and hold them in vesicles called endosomes. Many organisms trapped in endosomes are later destroyed by enzymes from lysosomes. *Leishmania* parasites, however, survive and multiply in the endosomes.

Fortunately, the body has a method for eliminating intracellular parasites sequestered in this way. Vertebrate organisms possess sets of molecules that bind to peptides produced within the cell and bring them to the cell surface, where they can be recognized by the immune system. These major histocompatibility complex (MHC) molecules have a groove in their structure that can bind to a range of antigenic peptides, or protein fragments. There are two classes of MHC molecules; in the case of *Leishmania* infections of macrophages, it is the class II MHC molecules that pick up peptides from the microbes (see boxed fig-ure "How the Immune System Fights *Leishmania*").

Class II MHC molecules are imported into the vacuoles containing the *Leishmania* organisms and other extracellular antigens ingested by the macrophage. The MHC molecules become loaded with peptides shed by the parasites or cleaved from them by the proteolytic enzymes. Not all the peptides present will be able to associate with the class II MHC molecules, but from an antigen as complex as *Leishmania*, at least several will. These complexes of MHC molecules and peptides then move to the macrophage's outer membrane.

Once displayed on the surface, the complexes can alert passing CD4 *T* cells to the presence of the intracellular infection. These *T* cells have receptor molecules that can recognize one particular peptide–class II MHC combination. All the receptors on a *T* cell are identical, as are those on *B* cells, but the great diversity of receptors made by the *T* cell population ensures that a match can be found for virtually any peptide-MHC combination. Thus, with the help of MHC molecules, *T* cells can recognize antigens from pathogens that hide inside cells.

This recognition event develops into an immunologic response if the macrophage also provides an additional signal to the *T* cell. One surface molecule that can provide this "accessory function" is B7, which macrophages and similar cells express when they become infected. B7 is recognized by a separate protein, CD28, on the *T* cell's surface. Interactions both between the *T* cell receptor and the peptide–class II complex and between B7 and CD28 are necessary for the CD4 *T* cells to mobilize an optimal response.

Indeed, in the absence of the accessory B7 signal, a CD4 *T* cell may become anergized, or inactivated, by its exposure to the antigenic peptide.

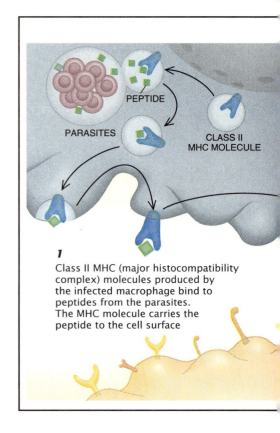

1

Class II MHC (major histocompatibility complex) molecules produced by the infected macrophage bind to peptides from the parasites. The MHC molecule carries the peptide to the cell surface

Thereafter, that cell may be unable to respond to the antigen. The induction of B7 expression on macrophages displaying foreign antigens seems to be very important for eliciting protective immune responses by CD4 *T* cells against intracellular pathogens.

When a CD4 *T* cell does receive the dual signal, it releases cytokines that increase the macrophage's ability to destroy the enemy within. The most critical of these cytokines, gamma-interferon, prompts the macrophage to produce other cytokines, such as tumor necrosis factor, and chemicals such as nitric oxide and toxic forms of oxygen, which lead to the microbe's destruction.

Studies have revealed, however, that the type of response by the CD4 *T* cells can vary, thereby significantly altering the efficacy of the protective reaction. Much of the detailed work on *Leishmania* infections has been conducted in mice, which are susceptible to the parasite *L. major*. In most strains of mice, experimental infections with *L. major* are transitory: the animals' immune system can purge few if any bacilli. The *T* cells of people who have tuberculoid leprosy vigorously produce gamma-interferon. In contrast, those with the severe lepromatous form of the disease have lesions containing vast numbers of intracellular bacilli; their immune responses are dominated by the production of interleukin-4.

Detailed investigations of such responses in tuberculosis patients have not yet been completed. It is nonetheless well known that most individuals can stave off the infections because their highly effective immune response prevents the tuberculosis bacilli from spreading beyond small lesions ringed by white blood cells. Only in a minority of patients does the disease progress and become fatal if left untreated. It is tempting to speculate that the outcomes of those infections may be determined in part by whether the response of their CD4 *T* cells is dominated by the release of protective gamma-interferon or of macrophage-incapacitating interleukin-4 and interleukin-10.

Insights from this work could someday be a boon to vaccine researchers. By blocking the effects of interleukin-4 at the time of inoculation, experimenters might be able to coax the antigen-challenged *T* cells to produce the protective

gamma-interferon. Experiments have shown that if susceptible mice receive an injection of monoclonal antibodies against interleukin-4 at the onset of a *Leishmania* infection, the animals can control the spread of the parasite. The monoclonal antibodies seem to neutralize the interleukin and allow the *T* cells to differentiate into gamma-interferon producers.

Conversely, when *Leishmania*-resistant strains of mice have been injected simultaneously with the parasite and interleukin-4, the animals develop more severe infections. Good vaccine strategies should therefore be aimed at maximizing the production of gamma-interferon at the time of immunization and either blocking or eliminating the action of interleukin-4. Recently the newly described cytokine interleukin-12 has been shown to increase strikingly the capacity of CD4 *T* cells to develop into gamma-interferon producers. The use of interleukin-12 in vaccines therefore deserves study.

Like many bacteria and parasites such as *Leishmania*, viruses establish infections inside the cells of the body, beyond the reach of antibodies. Unlike *Leishmania*, however, viruses live in the fluid interior of the cell and not inside a vacuole (see Figure 5.4). They interact freely with many cellular com-

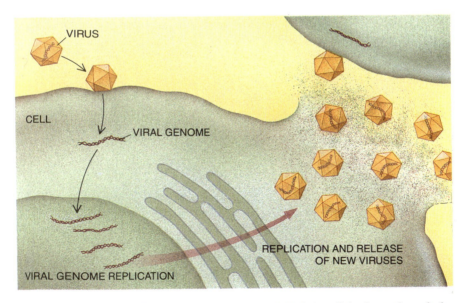

Figure 5.4 VIRUSES invade cells by binding to certain surface molecules and penetrating the membrane. Once within the cell, the viruses then use many components of the cell to replicate themselves. Cytopathic viruses damage and sometimes kill their cellular hosts through these processes. Immune defenses that are effective against other types of infections may not work against viruses.

How the Immune System Fights *Leishmania*

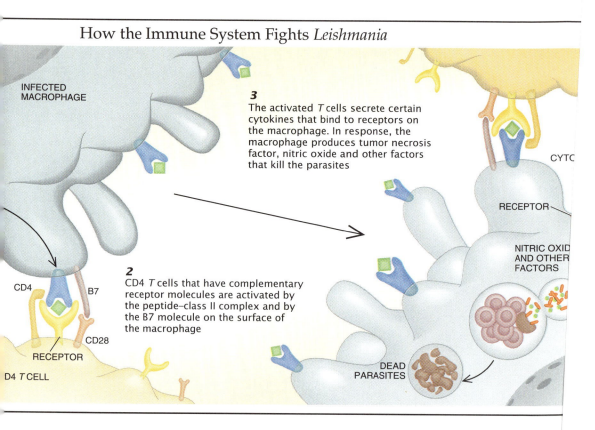

INFECTED MACROPHAGE

3
The activated *T* cells secrete certain cytokines that bind to receptors on the macrophage. In response, the macrophage produces tumor necrosis factor, nitric oxide and other factors that kill the parasites

CYT0

RECEPTOR

NITRIC OXID AND OTHER FACTORS

CD4

B7

2
CD4 *T* cells that have complementary receptor molecules are activated by the peptide–class II complex and by the B7 molecule on the surface of the macrophage

CD28

RECEPTOR

D4 *T* CELL

DEAD PARASITES

them. Their CD4 *T* cells, when activated by leishmanial antigens, produce gamma-interferon. Yet some inbred mice, such as those belonging to the BALB/c strain, cannot control *Leishmania* infections: instead they develop progressive lesions and eventually succumb. The reason for that failure seems to be that, when stimulated, their CD4 *T* cells predominantly secrete the cytokines called interleukin-4 and interleukin-10, and not gamma-interferon. The combination of those two interleukins is an especially powerful blocker of the microbe-killing activities that gamma-interferon induces.

Clearly, which cytokine the *T* cells "choose" to make in response to intracellular infection is critical to the course of the disease. Subsequent research has revealed details about how CD4 *T* cells make that decision. In general, when *T* cells in culture are exposed to antigenic peptides displayed on macrophages or other presenting cells, they are stimulated to develop into cells that can secrete large amounts of gamma-interferon and interleukin-2, a cytokine that prompts *T* cell prolifera-

tion, but little or no interleukin-4. leukin-4 is present in the growth me the *T* cells first recognize the display they produce more of that cytokine gamma-interferon. The choice betweer terleukin-4 or gamma-interferon seem a commitment by the lymphocyte. On *T* cell has responded to an antigen b one of these cytokines, it and its prog produce the other.

Those observations may partially the outcomes of some infectious di from one person to the next. *Leishma* ir humans take divergent courses. Mc able to control the parasite without be but in a few the infection develops in asis. Evidence now being collected differences in the patterns of cytoki by a patient's *T* cells may contribute t of the infections.

A similar divergence seems to be a rosy. In tuberculoid leprosy, the mild major forms of the disease, the skin l ponents. Viruses use the protein-synthesizing apparatus of human cells, for example, to manufacture their own proteins. Consequently, the viral proteins intermingle with the normal cellular proteins instead of staying within a neat vacuole bundle and so present a less easily isolated target for the molecules of the immune system.

Despite the intimacy of this arrangement, MHC molecules in all the body's cells can still find and display peptide fragments from viruses. The process is fundamentally similar to the one that reveals *Leishmania* infection, but it has some important differences (see boxed figure "How the Immune System Fights Viral Infections"). First, the MHC molecules that can bind to peptides from the cytosol are class I proteins, which differ in structure from the class II molecules. When viral and cellular proteins are fragmented in the cytosol, transporter molecules carry them into the organelle called the rough endoplasmic reticulum. There the peptides are loaded onto the class I MHC molecules. After further processing, the peptide–class I MHC complexes are shipped to the cell's surface in secretory vesicles. Once they are inserted into the outer membrane, the complexes can be examined by *T* cells. In this case, however, the lymphocytes are CD8 *T* cells, which bear receptors specific for the class I complexes.

When CD8 *T* lymphocytes detect antigenic peptides, they often act, directly and indirectly, to kill the infected cells. These *T* cells can destroy their infected targets by secreting perforin and other proteins that disrupt the integrity of the cellular membrane. Recent work indicates that the killer *T* cells may also act by producing molecules that elicit a form of cell death called apoptosis—in effect, these signals tell the infected cell that it should kill itself. In addition, activated CD8 cells release potent cytokines, including gamma-interferon and tumor necrosis factor. Those molecules limit viral replication inside a cell, while also attracting macrophages and other phagocytes that can destroy the cell.

The control of viral infections through the destruction of the body's own cells has some powerful advantages. If the recruitment of antigenic peptides by the class I MHC molecules and the subsequent *T* cell response are fast enough, the infected cells can be destroyed even before the viral particles inside them have been completely assembled. Any virus particles that may be released when the cells are killed will not be capable of in-

fecting other cells, and so the infection will be terminated before it can propagate.

On the other hand, the immunologic response mediated by CD8 *T* cells carries the potential for extensive harm to the host. If a virus multiplies and radiates quickly, the immune system's attempts to contain it may do no more than leave a path of destruction in the wake of the virus, while never quite catching up to it. The tissue damage associated with the infection would therefore result from the effects of both the virus and the immune reaction. In general, the amount of tissue damage caused by such an infection will be largely determined by how fast the immune response occurs in relation to the rate of spread of the virus.

The antiviral immune response becomes even more problematic when the viral infection itself does little or no damage to the cells—and many viruses do indeed infect cells without seriously impairing cellular function. Such noncytopathic infections can still provoke forceful reactions by CD8 cells. If the harmless virus spreads relatively quickly, the *T* cells may end up attacking a very large number of the host's cells. In these cases, the disease stems not from the virus at all but rather from the immune response.

One experimental demonstration of the harm that such immune responses can do comes from work with the lymphocytic choriomeningitis virus (LCMV), which infects tissues in the nervous system but has relatively little intrinsic pathogenicity. If newborn mice are inoculated with LCMV, the infection disperses speedily through their tissues but causes no evident disease. The reason is that their immature immune systems learn to tolerate the viral antigens as harmless constituents of the body; consequently, their *T* lymphocytes ignore the LCMV-infected cells. If cytotoxic *T* cells that respond to LCMV antigens are injected into these mice, however, the immune response is drastic and often kills the animals.

A variety of noncytopathic human infections show a similar pattern of tissue injury. Chronic carriers of the hepatitis *B* virus, for example, typically suffer liver damage even though it is a fairly harmless pathogen. The destruction of the infected liver cells is almost certainly a consequence of actions waged by cytotoxic *T* cells, which can be found in both the blood and the liver of the patients.

There are indications that the immune system

How the Immune System Fights Viral Infections

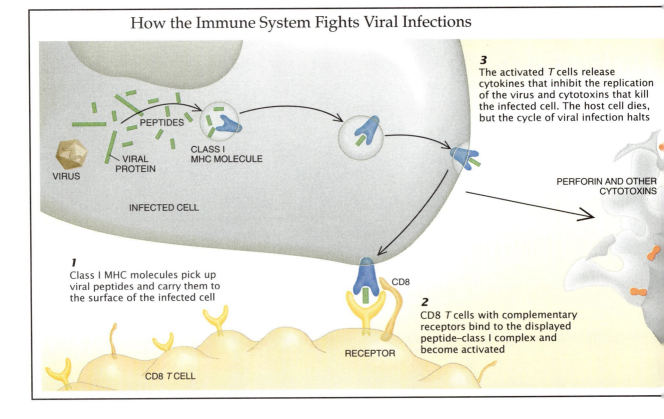

3 The activated *T* cells release cytokines that inhibit the replication of the virus and cytotoxins that kill the infected cell. The host cell dies, but the cycle of viral infection halts

PEPTIDES

CLASS I MHC MOLECULE

VIRAL PROTEIN

VIRUS

INFECTED CELL

PERFORIN AND OTHER CYTOTOXINS

1 Class I MHC molecules pick up viral peptides and carry them to the surface of the infected cell

CD8

2 CD8 *T* cells with complementary receptors bind to the displayed peptide–class I complex and become activated

RECEPTOR

CD8 *T* CELL

---

may sometimes subvert its own reaction to viral infections if that response would hurt the host more than the pathogen. Investigators have shown that if mice are injected with overwhelming numbers of LCMV, the CD8 *T* cells that should mobilize against the infection become activated but then die. Indeed, it seems likely that such cell deaths are the common result of a highly exuberant *T* cell response to an antigenic stimulus.

The elimination of those antigen-specific *T* cells leaves a strategic hole in the immunologic defense. Against a noncytopathic virus, this deficiency may be to the host's benefit because it allows the cells harboring the virus to survive. One might argue that the elimination of these *T* cells after an exposure to overwhelming numbers of a virus is an adaptation of the immune system to an infection that it cannot control without causing irreparable injury to the host. As long as the persistence of the virus does not lead to the death of its host cells or to malignant abnormalities, the lack of an answering immune response will protect against disease.

Such examples illustrate the fallibility of this elegant but imperfect defense system: the very mechanisms that provide protection against certain kinds of disease will sometimes abet the pathology of others. Perhaps the cruelest demonstration of this principle comes from viral infections that exploit the cells and interactions of the immune system to propagate themselves. In such infections the immune response actually assists the replication of the virus rather than limiting it.

That is exactly what happens when people become infected by the human immunodeficiency virus (HIV) that causes AIDS. The virus resides preferentially in CD4 *T* lymphocytes and other cells of the immune system. As it turns out, activated *T* cells are much more hospitable to growing viruses than are resting *T* cells; consequently, the more agitated the immune system becomes, the better the conditions for viral replication. In addition, cytokines such as tumor necrosis factor, which *T* cells produce when they detect viral anti-

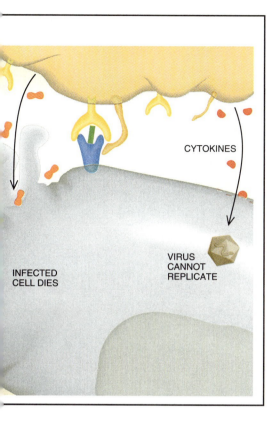

CYTOKINES

INFECTED
CELL DIES

VIRUS
CANNOT
REPLICATE

gens, can actually stimulate the replication of viruses in CD4 *T* cells. Thus, HIV uses the most sophisticated defenses of the immune system to further its own survival.

Diseases such as AIDS are a painful reminder of the challenges that pathogens continue to pose to human immunity. The tremendous diversity and mutability of infectious agents ensure that such challenges will not abate. Nevertheless, the understanding of the molecular basis of cellular responses is developing rapidly and promises to illuminate new ways to minimize tissue damage and to control infection. Harnessing our knowledge to boost immune responses will be critical to efforts to conquer the present and future microbial threats to humanity.

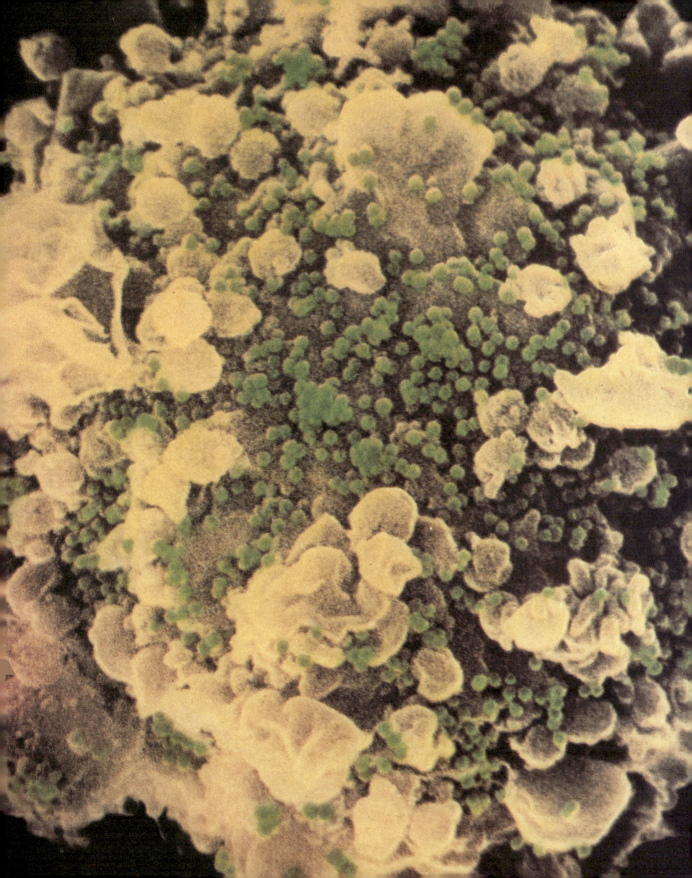

AIDS and the Immune System

The AIDS virus exploits the immune system to replicate itself. New findings are showing how it wreaks havoc on the body's defenses.

• • •

Warner C. Greene

It is now 12 years since acquired immunodeficiency syndrome sprang into medical and public awareness as a fatal disease of the immune system. The term "AIDS," or its equivalent in other languages, has since become recognized around the world. Other illnesses besides AIDS cause inappropriate immune responses, as numerous examples in this book illustrate. Yet AIDS warrants special consideration.

First, it is now tragically clear that the virus that causes AIDS, the human immunodeficiency virus (HIV), is one of the principal threats to human life and health worldwide. In an article about the epidemiology of AIDS published in SCIENTIFIC AMERICAN in October 1988, Jonathan M. Mann, James Chin, Peter Piot and Thomas Quinn estimated that more than 250,000 cases of the disease had then occurred worldwide and that between five and 10 million people were infected with HIV. Five years later the situation is far worse.

The Global AIDS Policy Coalition, which Mann coordinates, now estimates that the actual number infected by the end of 1987 was about seven million; it places the number infected by the end of 1992 at 19.5 million, almost three times the earlier figure. Although antiviral and other medications may modestly prolong the lives of those infected, the great majority of them will, barring some major advance, eventually die of an AIDS-related illness. More than three million people have developed full-blown AIDS; most have already died. Responsible estimates of the number of cases of HIV infection likely to have occurred by the year 2000 range from 40 million to more than 110 million. The second number is about 2 percent of the world's present population.

To be certain, other diseases, such as malaria, kill more people than AIDS does. But the rapid spread of HIV, together with the lack of a vaccine or satisfactory treatment, makes this disease uniquely alarming. New infections—the majority now from heterosexual contact—continue at the estimated rate of one every 15 seconds. No country or social group is immune. Currently HIV is spreading quickly in East Asia, a region that was largely spared in the early years of the pandemic. Worldwide, women now account for some 40 percent of AIDS cases; about 10 percent are children born to infected mothers. Public education campaigns aimed at reducing transmission—mainly exhortations to the sexually active to use condoms and to drug users to sterilize needles and syringes—have had limited success.

Figure 6.1 *T* LYMPHOCYTE infected with the human immunodeficiency virus (HIV) displays a characteristic lumpy appearance. The protuberances colored green in this electron photomicrograph are virus particles in the process of budding.

The second reason for discussing HIV is that it is the most intensively studied virus in history. We already have an outline sketch of how the genes and proteins in the HIV virion, or virus particle, operate. We still lack, however, a clear understanding of what controls its replication and how it destroys the human immune system.

I must emphasize that all responsible opinion holds that HIV is indeed the primary cause of AIDS. A small number of cases of people with immune deficiency who are not infected with HIV received inappropriately widespread publicity in 1992, which fostered the unsubstantiated notion that there is another cause of AIDS not detected by current blood tests. This unfortunate episode only fueled the paranoia that surrounds the disease. In fact, there is little reason to believe that the condition of these patients was caused by any virus or that it is becoming more common.

Yet there are many different strains of HIV, and epidemiological and laboratory studies suggest that some are deadlier than others. HIV-2, for example, which is prevalent in West Africa, seems to produce less severe disease than does HIV-1, the more common form elsewhere. It is even possible that some rare strains are benign. Some homosexual men in the U.S. who have been infected with HIV for at least 11 years show as yet no signs of damage to their immune systems. My colleagues Susan P. Buchbinder, Mark B. Feinberg and Bruce D. Walker and I are studying these long-term survivors to ascertain whether something unusual about their immune systems explains their response or whether they carry an avirulent strain of the virus.

The great majority of investigators believe not only that HIV is the primary cause of AIDS but also that HIV infection alone will usually cause profound immune dysfunction over time. No other specific pathogen is known to be necessary. It does seem likely that other infections in a person carrying HIV may hasten immune deficiency; this area is being actively investigated. Such opportunistic infections, which frequently complicate the clinical course of HIV-infected patients, are often the eventual cause of death. Nevertheless, if we are to understand AIDS, we must understand HIV.

High-resolution electron microscopy has shown the HIV virion to be roughly spherical and about one ten-thousandth of a millimeter across (see Figure 6.1). Its outer coat, or envelope, consists of a double layer of lipid molecules similar to and taken from the membranes surrounding human cells. This bilayer is studded with proteins, including some of human origin. These proteins, the so-called class I and class II major histocompatibility complex molecules, are, in their normal location, important in controlling the immune response.

The coat of the virion also bears numerous viral protein "spikes" that project into the external medium (see Figure 6.2). Each spike probably consists of four molecules of a protein called gp120 on the outside and the same number of gp41 embedded in the membrane. (Gp stands for glycoprotein— the proteins are linked to sugars—and the number refers to the mass of the protein, in thousands of daltons.) These envelope proteins play a crucial role when HIV binds to and enters target cells.

Underneath the envelope is a layer of matrix protein called p17, which in turn surrounds the core, or capsid. It has the shape of a hollow, truncated cone made of another protein, p24, which contains the genetic material of the virus. Because HIV is a retrovirus, its genetic material is in the form of RNA, or ribonucleic acid, rather than the more usual DNA, or deoxyribonucleic acid. Two strands of RNA, about 9,200 nucleotide bases long, fit within the viral core. They are attached to molecules of an enzyme, reverse transcriptase, which transcribes the viral RNA into DNA once the virus has entered a cell. Also present with the RNA are an integrase, a protease and a ribonuclease, enzymes whose functions I shall describe later. Two other proteins, p6 and p7, are present as well.

The gp120 envelope protein can bind tightly to CD4, a protein found in the membranes of several types of immune system cells. This property makes such cells vulnerable to HIV infection. When the gp120 of a virion binds to a cell bearing CD4, the membranes of the virus and the cell fuse, a process governed by the gp41 envelope protein. The virus core and its contents are then brought inside the cell.

Some CD4-bearing cells, known as dendritic cells, are present throughout the body's mucosal surfaces and elsewhere; it is possible that these are the first cells infected by HIV in sexual transmission. Immune system cells called macrophages and monocytes also carry the CD4 molecule and are similarly vulnerable. Macrophages, in particular, may carry HIV to other parts of the body,

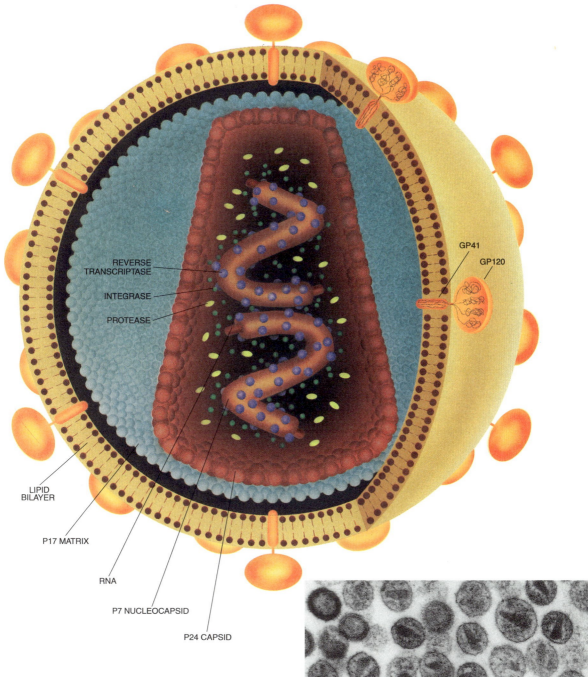

REVERSE
TRANSCRIPTASE

INTEGRASE

PROTEASE

GP41

GP120

LIPID
BILAYER

P17 MATRIX

RNA

P7 NUCLEOCAPSID

P24 CAPSID

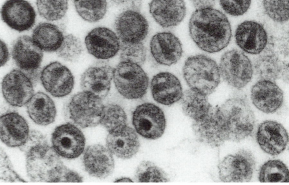

Figure 6.2 ANATOMY OF HIV: electron microscopy and other techniques have led to a consensus on the complex structure of the AIDS virus (above). The truncated cone-shaped core in a spherical envelope is the dominant feature. The micrograph (right) shows HIV particles in an intracellular space inside a cultured human macrophage. Cores can be discerned in mature virions; they are lacking in immature virus particles.

including the brain. But HIV's principal targets are the CD4-bearing helper *T* lymphocytes, or *T*4 cells. These cells help to activate other components of the immune system, particularly killer *T* cells (which attack virus-infected cells) and *B* cells (which produce antibodies).

Once an HIV virion has entered a cell, a complex sequence of events follows that, if completed, leads to the budding of new virus particles from the infected cell. But when a person acquires an HIV infection, he or she initially mounts a vigorous immune defense. During this acute phase of the infection, *B* cells produce antibodies that neutralize the virus, and activated killer *T* cells multiply and destroy infected cells, much as they would in many other diseases. Although it is possible that the immune system may successfully fight off HIV at a very early stage, by the time antibodies to HIV are found in the blood, infection is generally permanent.

The clinical picture in acute HIV infection is that of a mild, flulike illness, typically with fever and muscle aches, that usually lasts no more than a few weeks. During this time, large amounts of the virus are present in the bloodstream, and transmission is probably relatively easy. Then the immune response is mounted and begins to eliminate infected cells and circulating viruses. A proportion of infected cells remains, however, eluding the host's defenses, and the virus continues to replicate in lower numbers for as long as a decade. For most of this period of chronic infection, the patient is usually quite well. Only after several years does the virus so significantly damage the immune system that opportunistic malignancies and infections appear.

Ideas about how the damage takes place have shifted considerably in the past two years. When Michael S. Gottlieb of the University of California at Los Angeles first described in 1981 the clinical syndrome that came to be known as AIDS, he noted that his patients had very low numbers of *T*4 lymphocytes in their blood. Studies have since demonstrated that these cells decrease gradually in number during the long subclinical phase of chronic infection, from about 1,000 per cubic millimeter to less than 100. The observation naturally suggested that the decrease in *T*4 cells was responsible for the decline in immune function that happens over the same period.

For a while, it seemed possible that HIV causes the decrease in numbers of *T*4 cells solely by infecting and killing them. Most researchers now believe the process is more complex. Even in patients in the late stages of HIV infection with very low blood *T*4 cell counts, the proportion of those cells that are producing HIV is tiny—about one in 40. In the early stages of chronic infection, fewer than one in 10,000 *T*4 cells in blood are doing so. If the virus were killing the cells just by directly infecting them, it would almost certainly have to infect a much larger fraction at any one time.

Another clue that a more complicated process is involved comes from a recent experiment done by Donald E. Mosier and his colleagues at the Scripps Research Institute in La Jolla, Calif. They found that strains of HIV that kill *T*4 cells most effectively in culture are not necessarily those that cause the biggest depletion of *T*4 cells in genetically engineered mice that lack their own immune system and have been transfused with human CD4 cells.

If direct attack by the virus is not the only reason for the decline of *T*4 cells in blood, what are the other possibilities? A variety of plausible theories exist, although none has yet been proved, and indeed several different mechanisms may be at work. One theory is that uninfected killer *T* cells might start destroying infected immune system cells, including helper *T* cells. Other proposals are more complex. Antibodies that recognize gp120 and gp41 in the viral envelope might also attach to and interfere with histocompatibility antigens on healthy cells, impairing immune function. This could happen, some researchers have suggested, because gp120 and gp41 have characteristics similar to the histocompatibility antigens. Alternatively, those similarities could mean that gp120 triggers an immune attack on healthy *T*4 cells.

Another hypothesis rests on the fact that *T* cells are normally stimulated to divide when receptors on their surfaces recognize a foreign protein on another cell. Complexes of gp120 and gp41 that become detached from HIV, together with antibodies, may bind to the CD4 molecules on *T*4 cells and so prevent them from dividing, a phenomenon called anergy [see "T Cell Anergy," by Ronald H. Schwartz; SCIENTIFIC AMERICAN, August 1993].

Recent experiments point to yet another possibility. In people with HIV infection, many *T* cells—even those that are not infected—commit cellular suicide when they are stimulated by foreign proteins, rather than dividing as they should. This genetically controlled function, known as apoptosis, or programmed cell death, normally occurs in the thymus gland and serves to eliminate T cells that would attack the body's own tissues. But Joseph M. McCune and his colleagues at SyStemix have found evidence that HIV infection triggers widespread apoptosis in mice that, lacking an immune system, have had transplants of human fetal thymus and liver cells.

The researchers found that HIV caused a rapid loss of CD4 thymus cells in the implanted tissue, together with characteristic signs of apoptosis. A similar process might occur in infected humans. That could explain why AIDS progresses speedily in infants, whose immune systems are developing. The mechanisms that might trigger excessive apoptosis are, however, unknown.

Whatever the mechanisms, important clues have emerged about where much of the damage to the immune system is occurring. Researchers now know that $T4$ cells in the blood are not the main site of viral replication during the chronic asymptomatic phase of infection. Giuseppe Pantaleo and Anthony S. Fauci and their colleagues at the National Institute of Allergy and Infectious Diseases have shown convincing evidence that much of the

HIV is replicating not in the blood but in the scores of lymph nodes found throughout the body. The lymph nodes are where $T4$ cells, as well as other immune cells such as B cells, cluster to respond to foreign invaders.

Pantaleo and his associates have documented that HIV gradually destroys the lymph nodes (see Figure 6.3). The finding suggests that the decline in the number of $T4$ cells in the blood could be a result of damage to the lymph nodes. In fact, swelling of these organs has long been recognized as one early sign of infection. Nevertheless, for convenience, researchers have, perhaps mistakenly, usually focused on the changing cell counts and amounts of viral RNA—a marker for the virus—in the bloodstream.

The central involvement of the lymph nodes could explain one puzzling observation. During early chronic infection, the amount of viral RNA in the blood is very low. In fact, it is often impossible to detect by conventional techniques. As symptoms develop, the amount rises rapidly and may approach the peak levels present during the initial acute phase, prior to the immune response. A few investigators have surmised that some type of signal sets off a late wave of rapid

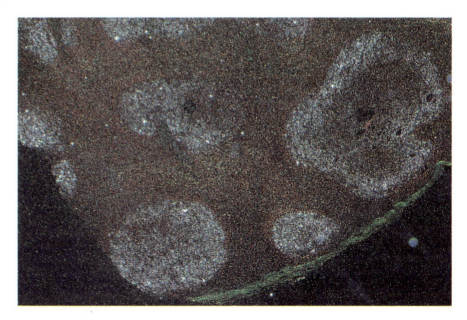

Figure 6.3 LYMPH NODES are believed to be an important site of HIV replication. In this section of a lymph node from a patient with early-stage infection, the tissue has been stained to show the presence of HIV (*white dots*) in localized patches.

viral replication that heralds the onset of full-blown AIDS. Recent technical advances in our ability to detect small amounts of the virus make this seem unlikely.

Rather it is now clear that the viral burden is substantial and increases steadily throughout most of the chronic asymptomatic phase of infection. The abrupt rise in blood levels of viral RNA in the last stages of infection can most likely be attributed to the "burning out" of the lymph nodes. These organs contain cells with delicate, fingerlike projections, known as follicular dendritic cells, that normally present antigens to T4 cells but also filter out various infectious agents. Collapsing nodes infected with HIV might no longer efficiently remove the virus, allowing its escape into the bloodstream. What precisely causes the death of the follicular dendritic cells remains a mystery, but the process may be as important as the loss of T4 cells.

Such thinking gains further support from the observation that even before a patient's T4 cells start to decline, a subset called memory T cells, which are responsible for remembering foreign proteins, begins responding abnormally to stimulation. Ultimately, these cells disappear. Other changes also occur. These phenomena could be a consequence of pathology in the lymph nodes.

The declining T4 cell count in the blood might, then, be at best an indirect indicator of damage taking place elsewhere in the body. If so, it underscores the importance of stopping the virus from multiplying even in the earliest stages of infection. One strategy being tried is to release "decoy" CD4 receptor molecules into the blood. These, it is reasoned, should attract HIV particles to stick to them rather than to CD4-bearing cells. Results so far have been disappointing, particularly against natural strains of the virus. It is likely that future

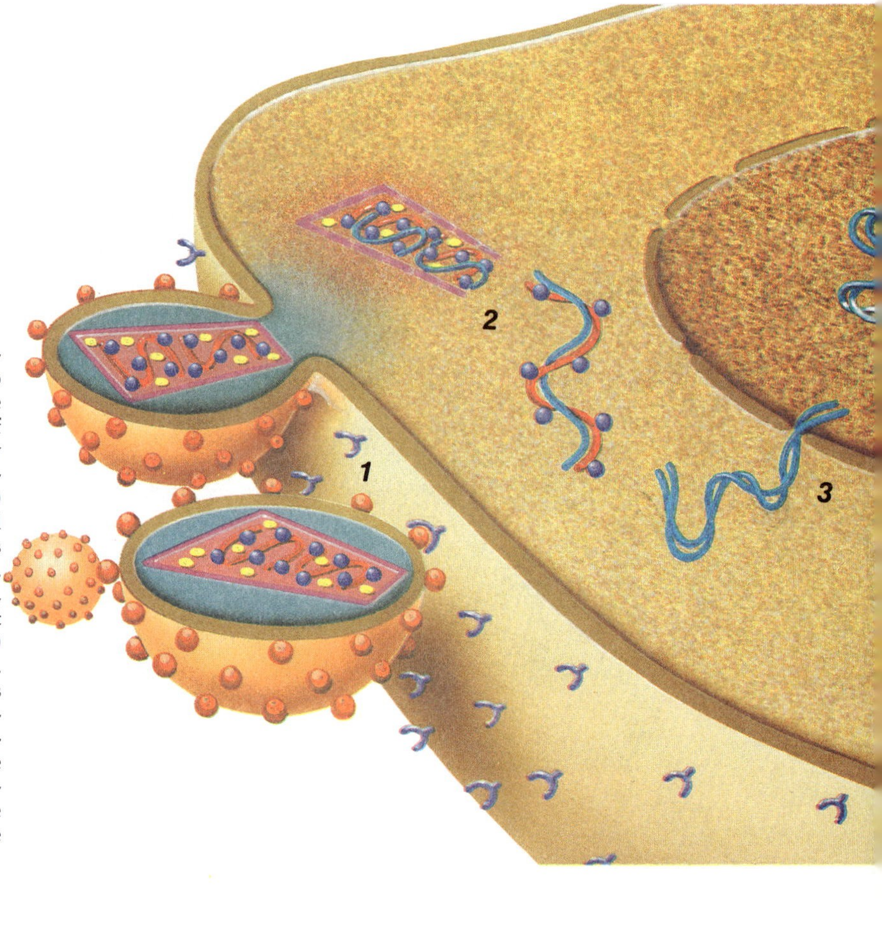

Figure 6.4 LIFE CYCLE OF HIV begins when virus particles attach to CD4 receptors on the cell membrane (1) and are drawn into the interior of the cell. The viral core then partially disintegrates (2) as reverse transcriptase (*purple*) produces DNA (*blue*) from the viral RNA (*red*). The viral DNA enters the nucleus, where it is integrated into host chromosomes (3). Host cell proteins bind to the DNA, initiating transcription (4). Short RNA molecules leave the nucleus (5) and make viral regulatory proteins. Later, medium-length and long RNAs leave the nucleus and generate structural and enzymatic proteins (6). Viral protease (*yellow*) becomes active as RNA and viral proteins (*orange*) enter the budding new virus (7). Core and other components form after the virus has budded (8).

interventions will focus on stopping the virus from replicating after it has entered a cell.

Thousands of meticulous experiments, many involving specially disabled strains of HIV, have demonstrated that inside a cell infected with HIV there is an intricate but elegant interplay among proteins produced by viral RNA and proteins produced normally in healthy cells. Significantly for the development of therapies, it is clear that only if the right conditions are met will HIV complete its life cycle and unleash scores of progeny that disseminate an infection.

The first thing that happens to the two strands of HIV RNA in a newly infected cell is that their encoded message is converted into DNA by the multiple reverse transcriptase molecules attached to the viral RNA. The process is the opposite of normal transcription, which makes RNA from DNA. Reverse transcriptase moves along the RNA, producing an equivalent chain of DNA by stitching

together the nucleotide building blocks. When the first DNA strand is completed, the reverse transcriptase starts constructing a second DNA strand, using the first one as a template (see Figure 6.4).

The reverse transcriptase that HIV uses is not very accurate: on average it introduces an error, or mutation, approximately once in every 2,000 incorporated nucleotides. This intrinsic infidelity underlies HIV's remarkable ability to become resistant to various drugs, because new variants of viral proteins are being constantly generated during the course of an infection.

The antiviral drugs that have been approved in the U.S. for treatment of HIV infection—azidothymidine (also known as AZT or zidovudine), dideoxycytidine (ddC) and dideoxyinosine (ddI)—all work by interfering with reverse transcription. Each is somewhat similar to one of the four nucleotides that reverse transcriptase connects together to build DNA. When the enzyme incorpo-

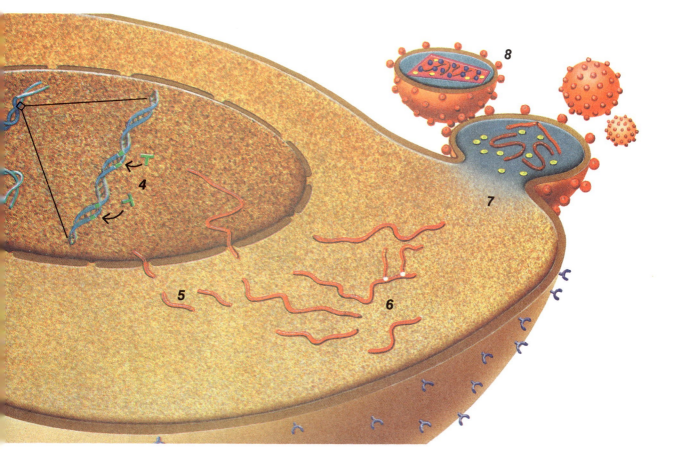

rates one of these drugs rather than a genuine nucleotide into a growing DNA strand, the reverse transcriptase cannot extend it further.

The problem is that the high rate of mutation means that within months variant reverse transcriptases appear in the body that can produce viral DNA even in the presence of the drugs. This rapid Darwinian evolution occurring within patients, as well as the toxicity of the drugs, almost certainly explains why the benefits of AZT are only temporary.

Other potential therapies aimed at blocking reverse transcriptase are on the horizon. One of these is the "convergent triple therapy" devised by Yung-Kang Chow and his colleagues at Harvard Medical School. These researchers had reported in *Nature* that the mutations reverse transcriptase undergoes in the presence of a mixture of AZT, dideoxyinosine and one other drug, nevirapine or pyridinone, are so extreme that the enzyme becomes ineffective. The workers have since found a flaw in their study, although clinical trials are proceeding. I suspect, however, that HIV will not easily succumb to drugs that are aimed at a single step in its life cycle.

Recent discoveries indicate other ways in which the early stages of viral replication might be thwarted. Irvin S. Y. Chen and his colleagues at the U.C.L.A. School of Medicine have performed experiments indicating that reverse transcription cannot be completed unless the host *T* cell is activated by a foreign protein. Other results, from Mario Stevenson and his co-workers at the University of Nebraska Medical Center, suggest that it is the next stage in the replication process that is blocked in resting cells. In this operation, the two DNA strands produced by reverse transcriptase are integrated into the host cell's chromosomes by the integrase present in the HIV virion.

In either case, the remarkable implication is that something made in a *T*4 cell when it is activated is critical to the virus's becoming integrated in the host cell. When unintegrated, HIV is unstable in the cell, decaying after a few days. That could be a weakness worth exploiting. Various immunosuppressive drugs, such as cyclosporine and FK 506, reduce the activation of *T* cells. A treatment protocol that intermittently decreased *T* cell activation might prevent HIV from being integrated and so prolong the asymptomatic phase of infection. Such an approach would not be without risk, since we know that a functioning immune system is vital for the initial containment of the virus. Experiments, perhaps employing monkeys infected with the HIV-like simian immunodeficiency virus (SIV), could delineate the relative benefits versus the dangers of the approach.

Once the two strands of HIV DNA have been integrated into the host cell's chromosomes, they are known as the provirus. As far as we can tell, infection of the cell is then permanent. But many processes still have to be completed before the cell can bud new virions. HIV is an extraordinarily complex virus. Whereas some retroviruses manage to get by with only three genes, HIV has nine or more, and at least five of them are essential for replication.

Before the provirus's genes can be effective, RNA copies of them that can be read by the host cell's protein-making machinery must be produced by forward transcription. This transcription stage is accomplished by the cell's own enzymes, including RNA polymerase II. But the process cannot start until the polymerase is activated by various molecular switches located in two stretches near the ends of the provirus: the long terminal repeats. This requirement is reminiscent of the need of many genes in multicellular organisms to be "turned on" by proteins that bind specifically to controlling sequences termed enhancer elements.

Some of the cellular signaling proteins that bind to the enhancers in the HIV long terminal repeats are members of an important family known as NF-κB/Rel. Present in virtually all human cells, these regulatory proteins increase the transcriptional activity of many genes. Significantly, cells step up production of some members of this family when they are stimulated by foreign proteins or by hormones that control the immune system. It appears that HIV utilizes the NF-κB/Rel proteins resulting from activation of immune cells to boost its own transcription.

The virus does not have everything its own way: my colleagues Stefan Doerre and Dean W. Ballard and I have found that one cellular protein, c-Rel, a member of the same NF-κB/Rel family, actually hinders HIV transcription. But it is made more slowly than are the factors that stimulate transcription. Clearly, the virus succeeds in getting itself transcribed often enough to spread infection. At first, the provirus relies on NF-κB and other proteins present in the activated cell to initiate its transcription into RNA. This process, though slow to begin with, can be likened to the tumbling of a stone that sets more and more stones rolling until it creates an avalanche.

The RNA transcripts from the provirus then undergo complex processing by enzymes in the cell. Two distinct phases of transcription follow the infection of an individual cell by HIV. In the early phase, which lasts roughly 24 hours, RNA transcripts produced in the cell's nucleus are snipped into multiple copies of shorter sequences by cellular splicing enzymes. When they reach the cytoplasm, they are only about 2,000 nucleotides in length. These early-phase short transcripts encode only the virus's regulatory proteins: the structural genes that constitute the rest of the genome are among the parts that are left behind (see Figure 6.5).

One of the first viral genes to be transcribed, *tat*, is encoded in the short transcripts and produces a regulatory protein that speeds up transcription of the HIV provirus. This protein acts by binding to a specific sequence within the viral RNA, called TAR. Once the tat protein binds to the TAR sequence, transcription of the provirus by cellular RNA polymerase II accelerates at least 1,000-fold. Ro 31-8959, a compound made by Hoffmann–La Roche, is in a new class of drugs that have the ability to inhibit the function of tat. It is now being evaluated in clinical trials.

Another regulatory gene expressed in the early phase is called *nef*. Until quite recently, it was believed that *nef*'s role was to suppress transcription, but new experiments have cast doubt on that interpretation. Nef protein may somehow modify the cell to make it more suitable for manufacturing HIV virions later. In any event, it now appears that production of nef protein is required for the development of AIDS, a finding that could be important if a way can be found to block its action.

A third regulatory protein encoded in the early short transcripts is called rev. We know that rev plays an essential role in the life cycle of HIV. Specifically, this protein appears to be responsible for switching the processing of viral RNA transcripts to the pattern that dominates once a cell has been infected for more than 24 hours. Rev protein binds to viral RNA at a sequence that is absent in the early short transcripts. Longer transcripts that do contain the rev-binding sequence are confined within the nucleus during the early phase. Once the amount of rev protein in the cell has built up to a high enough level, splicing and movement of the transcripts change to the pattern characteristic of the late phase.

In this late phase, two new size classes of RNA—long (unspliced) transcripts of about 9,200 bases and medium-length (singly spliced) transcripts of some 4,500 bases—move out of the nucleus and into the cytoplasm. These longer transcripts encode HIV's structural and enzymatic proteins. The crucial function of rev as a switch that turns on production of viral structural and enzymatic proteins makes it an attractive target for drug development. Unfortunately, no substance that effectively blocks rev's action has

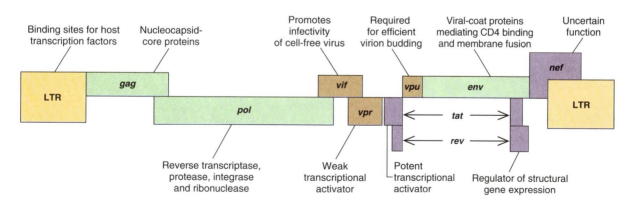

Figure 6.5 HIV GENES are indicated by the positions of colored bars along the DNA of the provirus. Genes that overlap utilize the same region of DNA but are read differently by protein-producing machinery of the host cell. Structural and enzymatic genes are green; regulatory genes, purple; others, tan. Sections called long terminal repeats (LTRs) are yellow.

yet been identified that is not unacceptably toxic.

Once the long and medium-length transcripts reach the cytoplasm, the cell's protein-making machinery begins constructing the components for new virions. The viral gene called *gag* encodes the core proteins; *pol* encodes the reverse transcriptase, protease, integrase and ribonuclease; and *env* encodes the two envelope proteins. Three other proteins encoded in the longer transcripts are produced as well, encoded by the *vpr*, *vif* and *vpu* genes. They have as yet ill-defined effects on infectivity, and the last two may play a part in the assembly of new virions. But all three seem to be significant for HIV's pathological properties.

The newly formed precursors of the proteins that will constitute the cores of new virions aggregate in the cytoplasm, together with complete copies of the viral RNA and the precursors of its associated enzymes. They all then move to the surface of the cell and bud through the membrane, where they acquire their lipid membranes and viral envelope proteins. During this final stage of assembly, the viral protease becomes active, cutting up the precursors to complete the core proteins and the enzymes. The structure of the protease, like that of the reverse transcriptase, is known in detail, and drugs have been designed to thwart its action. Trials of HIV protease inhibitors are under way at several clinical centers; results should be available within a few months.

Hope for the future should be tempered by the recognition that it is still true in 1993, as it was five years ago, that no satisfactory treatment for AIDS is yet in sight. Nevertheless, I am encouraged by how much we have learned in the past 12 years, and I believe that by the end of the second decade of the epidemic we will have antiviral therapies substantially better than those now available. I strongly suspect that these will consist of combinations of drugs directed against different parts of the life cycle of HIV.

In contrast, I feel there is less cause for optimism about prospects for the development of a practical prophylactic vaccine for HIV in the near future. The virus's ability to mutate quickly and by other means to elude immune responses poses a serious obstacle. Although clinical trials have shown that vaccines made from various viral proteins, chiefly the envelope, can improve human immune responses to the virus in laboratory tests, this is a far cry from demonstrating useful protection against natural infection. Even if a course of vaccinations could increase immunity, economic considerations may make such an approach unfeasible in the developing countries of the world where HIV is now spreading most rapidly.

There are some bright spots. Ronald C. Desrosiers of Harvard University and his colleagues have been able to make a vaccine that protects rhesus monkeys against infection from SIV. Desrosiers used as his vaccine a live strain of SIV that had its *nef* gene artificially disabled. The resulting virus establishes a persistent low-level infection that stimulates a strong immune response but causes no illness. Perhaps it will be possible to do something similar with HIV. Yet the safety problems surrounding the use of an attenuated but live HIV vaccine are daunting.

Even bolder approaches may find application in HIV therapy. One idea has been suggested by David Baltimore of the Rockefeller University, who shared a Nobel Prize in 1975 for discovering reverse transcriptase. Baltimore proposes introducing into an infected person's T cells a gene that would make the cells resistant to HIV infection. This approach, a form of gene therapy that Baltimore dubs "intracellular immunization," might be possible with the technology of the next century. Some mutant HIV genes that confer immunity on T cells in tissue culture have already been identified.

At present, we lack gene delivery and expression systems that could make such techniques widely applicable. If an injectable delivery system for protective genes could be developed, the approach might prove practical and cost-effective even in underdeveloped countries. This avenue merits investigation.

In the meantime, there is still much to be learned about HIV. For now, efforts to educate people about the virus should be redoubled. In the final analysis, preventing transmission of HIV is the best strategy.

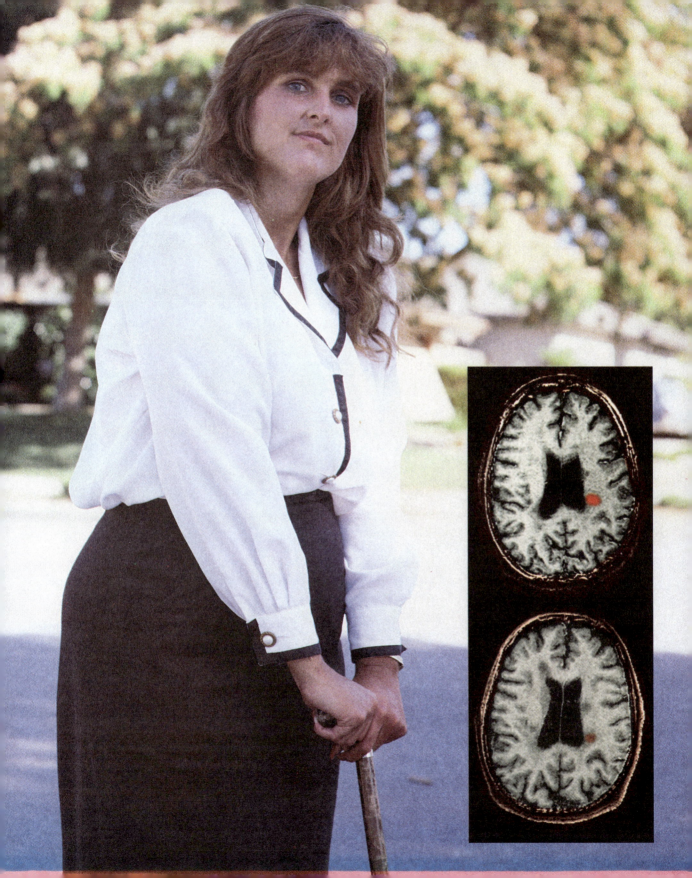

Autoimmune Disease

Misguided assaults on the self produce multiple sclerosis, juvenile diabetes and other chronic illnesses. Promising therapies are emerging.

• • •

Lawrence Steinman

Normally, the immune system is able to distinguish friend from foe, ignoring the body's own components and attacking foreign invaders. Unfortunately, the immunologic weapons can, like friendly fire, sometimes turn against the self, causing severe illness and even death.

Autoimmune diseases may involve any organ system, although some are affected more commonly than others: the white matter of the brain and spinal cord, in multiple sclerosis; the lining of joints, in rheumatoid arthritis; the insulin-secreting cells, in juvenile diabetes mellitus. Other forms of autoimmune disease ravage the connections between nerve and muscle in myasthenia gravis, stimulate the thyroid gland to produce excessive amounts of thyroid hormone in Graves' disease, blister the skin in pemphigus vulgaris or destroy the kidneys and other organs in a condition called systemic lupus erythematosus (see boxed figure "Where Autoimmunity May Strike").

Five percent of adults in Europe and North America—two thirds of them women—suffer from an autoimmune disease, many from more than one at a time. The affected population may turn out to be far larger if, as some workers suspect, autoimmunity plays an important secondary role in atherosclerosis, the cause of half the deaths in the Western world. Yet, if true, it might be good news, for science is making great strides in understanding autoimmunity.

In the past year, clinical trials have produced promising results for three experimental treatments of multiple sclerosis. Oral doses of myelin have induced tolerance for myelin proteins, and a genetically engineered monoclonal antibody as well as a naturally occurring substance—beta-interferon—has interrupted the process of inflammation, inhibiting relapses and thereby slowing the progression of disease. Small amounts of insulin, administered for the same purpose, have at least delayed and in some cases perhaps prevented the onset of diabetes in children at high risk for the disease. These findings suggest that advances in the treatment of one autoimmune disease may yield dividends for all the others.

The history of one of my patients, Kim Kent, reveals many aspects of autoimmune illness. She has multiple sclerosis, a disease that affects 250,000 Americans, two thirds of them women.

Kim is 26 years old and works as a travel agent in California. She first noted symptoms five years

Figure 7.1 KIM KENT has multiple sclerosis, a crippling disease in which the body's immune system attacks the white matter in the central nervous system. A characteristic lesion appears in a magnetic resonance image of Kim's brain (top). After treatment with an antibody against CD4—a molecule on the *T* cells that orchestrates the attacks—the inflammation subsided (bottom).

Where Autoimmunity May Strike

DISEASE	TARGET
Addison's disease	Adrenal gland
Autoimmune hemolytic anemia	Red blood cell membrane proteins
Crohn's disease	Gut
Goodpasture's syndrome	Kidney and lungs
Graves' disease	Thyroid
Hashimoto's thyroiditis	Thyroid
Idiopathic thrombocytopenic purpura	Platelets
Insulin-dependent diabetes mellitus	Pancreatic beta cells
Multiple sclerosis	Brain and spinal cord
Myasthenia gravis	Nerve/muscle synapses
Pemphigus vulgaris	Skin
Pernicious anemia	Gastric parietal cells
Poststreptococcal glomerulonephritis	Kidney
Psoriasis	Skin
Rheumatoid arthritis	Connective tissue
Scleroderma	Heart, lungs, gut, kidney
Sjögren's syndrome	Liver, kidney, brain, thyroid, salivary gland
Spontaneous infertility	Sperm
Systematic lupus erythematosus	DNA, platelets, other tissues

ago, when she felt tingling in her legs and pain in her arms. Her physicians diagnosed multiple sclerosis when a magnetic resonance scan revealed damage to the white matter, which contains the long nerve fibers that carry information to and from the brain. A year later she had a single episode of double vision, lasting about a week, and the year after that she began to have trouble keeping her balance while walking. She relied on a cane sometimes, particularly when tired. Her main problems now are poor balance, tingling in the legs and weakness of the right hand, which makes writing difficult.

In 1991 Kim began to participate in trials of a drug that eliminates a crucial actor in the autoimmune response. In the first month she received three intravenous infusions of a genetically engineered antibody to CD4, a molecule on certain T cells. More recently she has undergone therapy once every four months. As a result, the number of her CD4 T cells has declined far below the usual level. Yet other parts of the immune system con-

tinue to function normally, and Kim has developed no infections. Her symptoms have remained stable, with transient strengthening of her right hand and occasional periods of improvement in her walking. She now uses a cane only when walking outside her home. Her most recent magnetic resonance scan shows overall benefit, with noticeable regression in many lesions and clear evidence of repair of the white matter (see Figure 7.1). Some new lesions have also appeared, however.

As is the case with most autoimmune illnesses, genetic factors are evident: studies of monozygotic, or identical, twins show that when one twin gets multiple sclerosis, the other twin has about a 30 percent chance of acquiring it. The disease usually presents itself in early adulthood, often a few weeks after a routine illness. It also tends to flare after pregnancy. Periods of remission alternate with acute episodes of worsening in about half of the patients; in the remainder, the disease follows a continuously progressive course.

A picture of the cause of multiple sclerosis is at last coming into view. Self-reactive cells, which ought to be eliminated or silenced in the thymus gland during development, instead escape to the rest of the body. The thymus may fail to do its job because it does not come into contact with a sufficient quantity of self-antigens, particularly proteins that are ordinarily sequestered in a particular organ, such as the brain. The possibility also exists that the autoimmune response may be triggered by microbes that mimic the structure of self-antigens, especially if those antigens had not been presented to the thymus during development.

The self-reactive lymphocytes that are thus created migrate from the thymus, lymph nodes and spleen to the bloodstream and thence into the organs of the body, where they release chemicals that damage specific tissues. These insights have already suggested a number of ways in which the self-destructive cells might be removed or silenced.

Investigators had long wondered whether autoimmunity might be the cause of multiple sclerosis, but clear evidence came only in 1982, when Cedric S. Raine and his colleagues at the Albert Einstein College of Medicine in Bronx, N.Y., found immune cells in the white matter of patients. There they observed a pattern indistinguishable from simple inflammation: most of the immune cells were T lymphocytes, derived from the thymus; a few were B lymphocytes, derived from the bone marrow; the rest were scavenger cells, or macrophages. Each kind of cell plays a specific part in destroying the myelin sheath that insulates long nerve fibers, giving them their white coloration. It turns out, moreover, that the T and B cells achieve these ends by different means.

Two questions arose immediately: What were these cells doing to the white matter, and how did they penetrate the blood-brain barrier, which normally excludes agents of the immune system [see "Breaching the Blood-Brain Barrier," by Elaine Tuomanen; SCIENTIFIC AMERICAN, February 1993]. To answer the first question, researchers have extensively studied the T and B cells, in particular the structures, called receptors, with which they recognize antigen.

Analysis of the antigen receptor on B cells revealed that the spinal fluid of patients with multiple sclerosis had an increased content of antibody. Most of the antibody had been produced by just a few clones of B cells. In the early 1980s Claude

C. A. Bernard and his colleagues at La Trobe University in Australia demonstrated that some of the antibodies precipitated the destruction of the major constituent of the myelin sheath: myelin basic protein.

The B cells' antibodies attack not the protein itself but the oligodendroglial cells in which it is made. The assault begins when the antibodies combine with blood-borne enzymes known as complement to form so-called attack complexes. D. Alistair S. Compston and his associates at the University of Cambridge have found complexes containing five components of complement in the cerebrospinal fluid of multiple sclerosis patients. The complexes fasten specifically to the membranes of oligodendroglial cells, where they interfere with the outward passage of calcium ions, thus destroying the cells.

The function of the T cells was more difficult to elucidate because, unlike antibody, they recognize a target—a peptide, or protein fragment—only when it is bound in a strategic pocket of one of the proteins referred to as human lymphocyte antigen, or HLA. (Such proteins sit on the membrane of the cell, presenting antigens to T cells for the same reason soldiers give passwords: to avoid being treated as an enemy.) A problem arises here because HLA molecules are not normally expressed in an appreciable manner within the nervous system. In multiple sclerosis, however, they are induced in the white matter by the cytokine gamma-interferon, one of the chemical signals through which immune system cells communicate.

Physicians discovered this connection by accident, while testing gamma-interferon as a therapy for multiple sclerosis. Instead of helping, the drug made matters worse by causing recurrent paralysis, and the clinical trial was stopped. Yet the results were instructive. They showed that viral infection and other stresses might aggravate the disease by eliciting the secretion of gamma-interferon in the brain. HLA molecules then appear in the cells of this region, where they are not normally expressed.

In 1983 Gian Franco Bottazzo of Middlesex Hospital Medical School and Marc Feldmann of University College, London, documented this process for the brain, in multiple sclerosis; the joint lining, in rheumatoid arthritis; and the pancreas, in juvenile diabetes. Such aberrant expression of HLA molecules explained how gamma-interferon worsened multiple sclerosis. It also provided a rationale for further experimental therapies using agents that blocked the expression of HLA at the sites of autoimmune disease.

Before such therapies could be designed, however, it was necessary to identify what the T cells were attacking in the white matter. To do so, researchers had to infer the structure of the T cell receptor from the sequence of genes that encode it. Unlike other genes, however, those for the T cell receptor rearrange themselves with respect to the order inherited on the chromosomes. It is therefore necessary to extract and analyze genes from the individual T cells—a daunting task until the mid-1980s, when a researcher at Cetus Corporation (now Roche Molecular Systems) developed a powerful technique of gene amplification known as the polymerase chain reaction [see "The Unusual Origin of the Polymerase Chain Reaction," by Kary B. Mullis; SCIENTIFIC AMERICAN, April 1990].

This technique proved invaluable to a team consisting of Bernard, Jorge R. Oksenberg, Michael A. Panzara and me at the Stanford University School of Medicine and Ann B. Begovich and Henry A. Erlich of Cetus Corporation. From 1989 to 1992, we analyzed RNA from lymphocytes at sites of inflammation in the brains of patients with multiple sclerosis. By sequencing a major set of T cell receptors, we were able to infer the receptors' target: the antigen complex formed when a particular fragment of myelin basic protein binds to a specific part of the HLA receptor—its DR2 molecule. We also found a sequence of three amino acids in the receptor that seemed to bind to the antigen complex.

Independent work conducted at the same time by Daniel P. Gold of the San Diego Regional Cancer Center and by Halina Offner-Vandenbark and Arthur A. Vandenbark of the Oregon Health Sciences University School of Medicine provided another crucial step. The researchers found the same, rearranged T cell receptor gene, the same amino acid triplet at the binding site and the same fragment of myelin basic protein in an animal model of multiple sclerosis called experimental allergic encephalomyelitis (EAE). These results were significant because they proved the value of the model, which is induced by autoimmunizing animals against myelin basic protein and which produces the clinical symptoms of multiple sclerosis: paralysis and demyelination. The model can thus test therapies for the human illness.

What turns the T cells against the self? Infection often precedes the onset of autoimmune disease, and so scientists have closely scrutinized the tactics that pathogens commonly employ to elude T cells. The answer appears to lie in molecular mimicry, an evolutionary adaptation whereby viruses and bacteria attempt to fool the body into granting them free access. Such mimicry works by showing the immune system stretches of amino acids that look like self. For example, adenovirus type 2 has amino acid sequences like those in the crucial fragment of myelin basic protein. In responding routinely to this virus, the immune system may become primed to attack the corresponding self-component—myelin.

An autoimmune response can begin even if the molecular mimicry is not quite exact. Anand Gautam and Hugh O. McDevitt of Stanford were able to induce paralysis in mice by exposing them to a short stretch of 10 amino acids, of which only five were actually identical to myelin basic protein. Robert S. Fujinami and Michael B. A. Oldstone of the Scripps Research Institute demonstrated that hepatitis B virus polymerase shared a stretch of just six amino acids with a part of the myelin basic protein molecule that causes EAE in rabbits. When they immunized rabbits with this part of the virus, the animals developed inflammation in their brains.

This research suggests that molecular mimicry between viruses or bacteria and self may be critical in initiating autoimmune responses. Scarring of the heart valves in rheumatic fever may be a consequence of the cross-reaction between myosin and a component of the cell-wall M protein in hemolytic streptococcal bacteria. Inflammation of the joints in rodents can be induced by immunization with Mycobacterium tuberculosis. This disease resembles rheumatoid arthritis and may arise from the similarities in structure between a core protein of cartilage and tuberculosis.

Obviously, not everyone responding to adenovirus type 2 mounts an immune response to myelin basic protein and develops multiple sclerosis. The reason seems to rest for the most part with the differences in individuals' HLA types. The HLA molecules determine exactly which fragments of a pathogen are displayed on the cell surface for presentation to T cells. One individual's HLA structure may bind a self-mimicking fragment and present it to the immune system, whereas another's may bind a fragment unique to the pathogen that does not mimic self. In the latter case, the pathogen is attacked, but self-tolerance is not violated (see Figure 7.2).

People who carry HLA-DR4 are six times more likely than others to acquire rheumatoid arthritis. Those with HLA-DR2 are four times more likely to inherit multiple sclerosis than those without it. Juvenile diabetes mellitus affects 0.2 percent of the U.S. population, but it is about 20 times more common in those white persons who have the HLA-DR3 and HLA-DR4 genes.

Yet, as is the case in all the autoimmune diseases, the genes by themselves cannot cause the disease. Five percent of those who have juvenile diabetes lack the genes, and five percent of the healthy population carry both of them. Even the twins of persons with this disease acquire it only about 50 percent of the time. Systemic lupus erythematosus has also been associated with certain HLA types, although here the concordance rate in twins is only 25 percent. Some HLA types predispose to several autoimmune diseases, ex-

plaining why those with myasthenia gravis, for instance, have a 30 percent chance of acquiring Graves' disease as well.

Genes may also confer protection against autoimmune diseases. In 1987 McDevitt, John I. Bell and John A. Todd of Stanford observed that resistance to juvenile diabetes correlates with the presence of the amino acid aspartate at position 57 of the HLA-DQ beta chain—one of two structures in the HLA protein. Erlich made the same discovery independently. Interestingly, among the Japanese, most of whom have precisely this HLA character, the prevalence of juvenile diabetes is just 5 percent of that observed in the U.S. In contrast, HLA-DQ beta chains with serine, alanine or valine at position 57 are associated with a high risk for juvenile diabetes. These correlations between HLA and disease are partly a result of whether a certain HLA molecule can present a fragment of a pathogen that mimics a self-constituent.

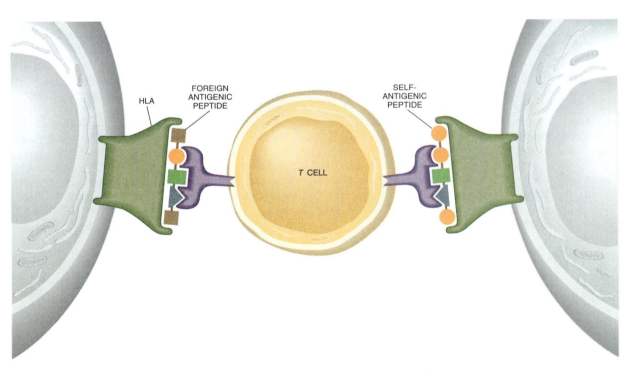

Figure 7.2 FRIEND OR FOE: *T* cells recognize foreign antigens when they are presented by the HLA molecules of the immune system. In some people, especially those who have certain HLA types, a foreign antigen may resemble antigen produced by the body. Such molecular mimicry provokes the *T* cells to attack body tissues that contain the self-antigens.

Autoimmunity, however it begins, must consist of more than the mere raising of an army of T cells: the cells must also travel from the thymus and spleen to the blood and thence to the target organ. Three categories of molecules are involved in this intricate homing mechanism. Movement through the blood vessel wall appears to be the same in autoimmune disease as in the normal inflammatory response to infection. The process of homing in on the target is mediated by members of the immunoglobulin supergene family and the T cell receptor, CD4 and CD8 (see Chapter 3, "How the Immune System Recognizes Invaders," by Charles A. Janeway, Jr.).

Here is how the process works. Once they arrive at the target, leukocytes—mainly T cells—get a foothold with the help of intracellular adhesion molecules called integrins. These molecules, which sit on the T cells, bear receptors that can be likened to Velcro fasteners. Counter receptors belonging to the immunoglobulin supergene family constitute the other half of the Velcro bond. The counter receptors grow from the endothelial lining of blood vessels at points that have been exposed to such cytokines as gamma-interferon and tumor necrosis factor.

These cytokines are produced on the spot by activated T cells and macrophages. Therefore, when a T cell rolls down a blood vessel and meets a counter receptor, it sticks. The process of sticking causes the T cell to secrete proteases, enzymes that help to create a hole in the blood vessel and enable the T cell to tighten its cytoskeleton so that it can squeeze through the tiny hole. In this manner, leukocytes break through the blood-brain barrier to cause multiple sclerosis (see boxed figure "How Multiple Sclerosis Progresses), penetrate the synovial lining to cause rheumatoid arthritis and so on for all the other autoimmune diseases.

Destruction begins when a T cell encounters its antigen in the cleft of an HLA molecule and releases proteins and peptides, including tumor necrosis factor, a chemical relative called lymphotoxin and gamma-interferon. These chemicals have been identified as the proximate cause of demyelination. Macrophages then speed the process, partly by secreting tumor necrosis factor and partly by mounting a direct attack. Raine and John Prineas of the University of Medicine and Dentistry of New Jersey have shown that macrophages actually strip fragments of myelin from the sheath encasing the nerve axons (see Figure 7.3).

One might suppose that autoimmune disease, once started, would proceed without interruption. Yet in multiple sclerosis, rheumatoid arthritis, systemic lupus erythematosus and myasthenia gravis, periods of deterioration usually alternate with remission. In all these diseases the pattern of decline has been shown to correlate strongly with three factors in the environment: female hormones, infection and stress.

It has long been noted that auto-immune disease is generally worse in women than in men. Recently Howard S. Fox of Scripps adduced a reason. He has shown that the female hormone estrogen stimulates a DNA sequence that stimulates nearby genes, which in turn transcribe gamma-interferon. Estrogen thus promotes the production of gamma-interferon, which, as we have seen, helps to induce the autoimmune process.

Microorganisms clearly cannot worsen existing autoimmune disease in the same way that they induce it—molecular mimicry will not cause the body to be more sensitive to one of its own components than it already is. Some other microbial function must be culpable. Its nature was suggested by a study of EAE by Stefan Brocke and his colleagues at Stanford. When the workers administered staphylococcal enterotoxin B to mice that had recovered from EAE-induced paralysis, relapses occurred within 48 hours. Staphylococcal enterotoxin B belongs to the class of substances known as superantigens, so called because they activate T cells that would otherwise respond only to differing, specific antigens.

Because superantigens reactivate rogue T cells, they greatly intensify the inflammation. They have this broad effect because they bind to the T cell receptor at a point that lies outside the highly specific site that recognizes antigen [see "Superantigens in Human Disease," by Howard M. Johnson, Jeffry K. Russell and Carol H. Pontzer; SCIENTIFIC AMERICAN, April 1992].

Of course, only those T cells that are primed for a self-antigen will find their way to the target. Brian L. Kotzin and Philippa Marrack of the National Jewish Center for Immunology and Respiratory Medicine in Denver have shown, for instance, that certain T cells bearing a specific receptor are concentrated in the synovial fluid of patients who have rheumatoid arthritis. That concentration is mirrored by a corresponding depletion of the same T cells in the bloodstream. Kotzin and Marrack proposed that these autoimmune *T* cells were activated by superantigens, so that they attacked the lining of joints and then proliferated in the synovial tissues, where they were selected by an as yet undetermined specific antigen.

Stress—such as sickness or trauma—can worsen autoimmune disease by affecting two glands in the brain: the hypothalamus and the pituitary. They then secrete hormones that promote inflammation. In addition, nerves may play a role by directly innervating lymph glands and immune cells resident in the organs.

Inflammation stimulates the release of cytokines, which travel to the brain's glands and cause them to secrete corticotropin-releasing factor. This neuropeptide has two opposed effects: it heightens the activity of immune cells at the site of inflammation and at the same time stimulates the adrenal glands to produce glucocorticoids, which shut down inflammation. One can block the inflammatory effect of corticotropin-releasing factor by using drugs, such as antibodies, that bind to the factor, neutralizing it.

In multiple sclerosis, especially during infection, such cytokines as tumor necrosis factor and interleukin-1 may be produced within the brain itself by glial cells (which support the functioning of the neurons). These cytokines may be augmented with others produced outside the brain and ferried into it through certain critical points in the blood-brain barrier. (Such effects are crucial in the etiology of simple fever: infection causes macrophages to produce interleukin-1, which enters the hypothalamus through a breach in the blood-brain barrier in the preoptic area. There it triggers a rise in body temperature.)

The nerves' possible involvement in immunity has long been suspected, but hard evidence came only a few months ago. Richard D. Granstein and his colleagues at Massachusetts General Hospital were able to show that nerves can release certain neuropeptides in the skin, thereby influencing the vigor of the local immune response. This local regulation may figure in psoriasis—clearly an autoimmune disease—a condition that worsens when the patient becomes anxious.

So far research has concentrated on the hormonal pathways that link stress to autoimmune reactions. Recently Ronald L. Wilder and George P. Chrousos and their colleagues at the National Institutes of Health have demonstrated that corticotropin-releasing factor is present in the synovial fluid and tissues of patients with rheumatoid arthritis. They also showed that animals that fail to release enough corticotropin-releasing factor in response to stress are quite susceptible to experimentally induced arthritis. Gabriel S. Panayi of Guy's Hospital Medical School, University of London, has noted the same features in rheumatoid arthritis patients. These findings may provide a link between the well-known clinical observation that anxiety can worsen autoimmune disease.

If fear can produce relapses, then even the fear of a relapse may become a self-fulfilling prophecy. Indeed, uncertainty about the future is perhaps the most bitter aspect of autoimmune disease. Remissions may last for months or for years, disease may progress slowly or rapidly, complications beyond the primary autoimmune process may or may not ensue. Moreover, the chances of developing another autoimmune condition are much enhanced in those who already have one.

Some of these secondary conditions are fairly innocuous because they destroy tissues whose function can be replaced. Graves' disease, for instance, can be treated by removing the overactive thyroid gland and then supplying the missing hormone orally. Yet the corresponding therapy for juvenile diabetes—insulin injections—leaves something to be desired. Such injections cannot fully reproduce the finely graded secretion of the beta cells, which controls the metabolism of glucose with exquisite sensitivity. The glucose concentration in the blood therefore fluctuates excessively, exposing the diabetic to a heightened risk of vascular complications. (In June, a long-term study sponsored by the National Institute of Diabetes and Digestive and Kidney Diseases concluded that patients can prevent or delay complications by testing their blood frequently and making appropriate adjustments in diet and exercise and insulin dosage.)

No substitute exists, however, for the tissue attacked in myasthenia gravis: the acetylcholine receptor at the junction between nerves and muscle. Antibodies attack the junction, causing weakness and paralysis. Tolerance to the acetylcholine receptor is broken in the thymus gland, where the acetylcholine receptor is expressed. In about half of the patients the gland becomes enlarged, and it is standard practice to remove it—a procedure that often alleviates the disease, especially in young patients.

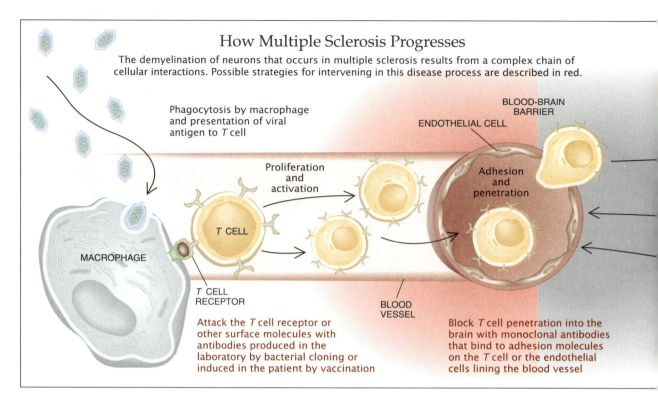

How Multiple Sclerosis Progresses

The demyelination of neurons that occurs in multiple sclerosis results from a complex chain of cellular interactions. Possible strategies for intervening in this disease process are described in red.

Phagocytosis by macrophage and presentation of viral antigen to *T* cell

BLOOD-BRAIN BARRIER

ENDOTHELIAL CELL

Proliferation and activation

Adhesion and penetration

T CELL

MACROPHAGE

T CELL RECEPTOR

BLOOD VESSEL

Attack the *T* cell receptor or other surface molecules with antibodies produced in the laboratory by bacterial cloning or induced in the patient by vaccination

Block *T* cell penetration into the brain with monoclonal antibodies that bind to adhesion molecules on the *T* cell or the endothelial cells lining the blood vessel

Systemic lupus erythematosus is perhaps the most devastating of the autoimmune diseases, capable of reaching virtually all the organs, sometimes one after the other, often with no warning at all. It affects about 250,000 people in the U.S., displaying an extraordinary imbalance in relation to sex: fully 90 percent of the patients are women. The illness generally begins in young adulthood when a characteristic skin rash appears over cheekbones and forehead, producing the wolflike impression from which the disease derives its name (see Figure 7.4). Hair loss is common, as is severe kidney damage, arthritis, accumulation of fluid around the heart and inflammation of the lining of the lungs. In nearly half of the patients the blood vessels of the brain also become inflamed, leading sometimes to paralysis and convulsions.

Why systemic lupus erythematosus is so protean remains a mystery, although the pathology in so many different tissues implies a general failure in self-tolerance. Recent experiments suggest an attractive explanation. Mice with a lupuslike disease turn out to have a mutation in the gene encoding *Fas*, a molecule found on the surface of thymocytes and on activated *T* and *B* cells. The normal *Fas* molecule triggers programmed death in immune cells. If the *Fas*-mediated death goes awry, self-reactive *T* and *B* cells of all kinds may wreak havoc in many different organ systems.

Until quite recently, physicians have had to fight these diseases in the dark, armed only with nonspecific immunosuppressants, such as the corticosteroids, which help very little and sometimes cause harm. In the past few years, however, our understanding of the pathogenesis of autoimmune disease has led to the development of highly selective therapies, each of which intervenes at a different point in the autoimmune process. These therapies have achieved excellent results in animal models, and some of them are undergoing clinical trials. Indeed, a few drugs are now awaiting approval.

If HLA molecules in the white matter are associated with attacks of multiple sclerosis, then it makes sense to block their expression. Beta-interferon has this blocking effect, just as gamma-inter-

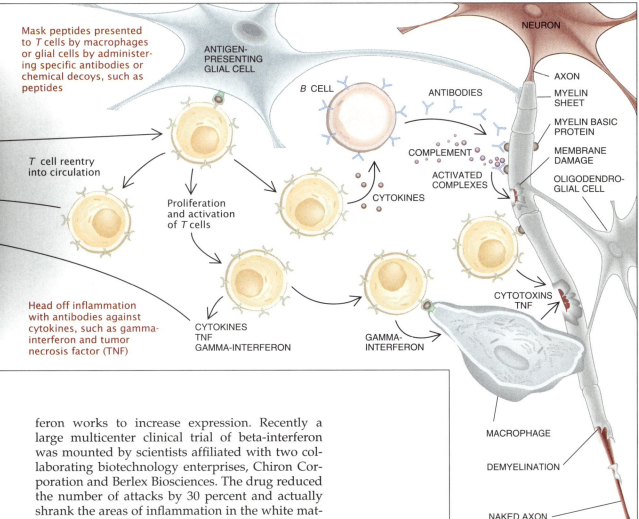

Mask peptides presented to T cells by macrophages or glial cells by administering specific antibodies or chemical decoys, such as peptides

NEURON

ANTIGEN-PRESENTING GLIAL CELL

B CELL

ANTIBODIES

AXON

MYELIN SHEET

MYELIN BASIC PROTEIN

COMPLEMENT

MEMBRANE DAMAGE

ACTIVATED COMPLEXES

OLIGODENDRO-GLIAL CELL

T cell reentry into circulation

CYTOKINES

Proliferation and activation of T cells

Head off inflammation with antibodies against cytokines, such as gamma-interferon and tumor necrosis factor (TNF)

CYTOKINES TNF GAMMA-INTERFERON

GAMMA-INTERFERON

CYTOTOXINS TNF

MACROPHAGE

DEMYELINATION

NAKED AXON

feron works to increase expression. Recently a large multicenter clinical trial of beta-interferon was mounted by scientists affiliated with two collaborating biotechnology enterprises, Chiron Corporation and Berlex Biosciences. The drug reduced the number of attacks by 30 percent and actually shrank the areas of inflammation in the white matter. In July the Food and Drug Administration recommended beta-interferon, making it the first approved therapy for multiple sclerosis.

Other strategies aimed at blocking the HLA molecules that present self-sensitive antigens may be even more direct and potent. In the animal model of multiple sclerosis, molecules similar to HLA-DR present fragments of myelin basic protein to T cells, which then attack the central nervous system. McDevitt and I and others showed that it is possible to make analogues of myelin that bind to the HLA molecules with higher affinity than the native myelin and yet are nonimmunogenic. By mopping up all the HLA molecules, the analogues serve as molecular decoys that prevent EAE and even reverse the associated paralytic disease.

Encouraged by these results, my colleagues at Neurocrine Biosciences (where I serve as chief scientist) are designing decoys that fit into the HLA cleft. They specifically turn off, or "tolerize," the T cells that destroy myelin. Neurocrine Biosciences holds the patent rights to this technology and is developing it, with my assistance, for clinical applications. There is reason to believe this strategy can be applied to all the autoimmune diseases. Michael Sela and Ruth Arnon and their colleagues at the Weizmann Institute of Science in Israel have synthesized a copolymer that resembles myelin basic protein. This copolymer

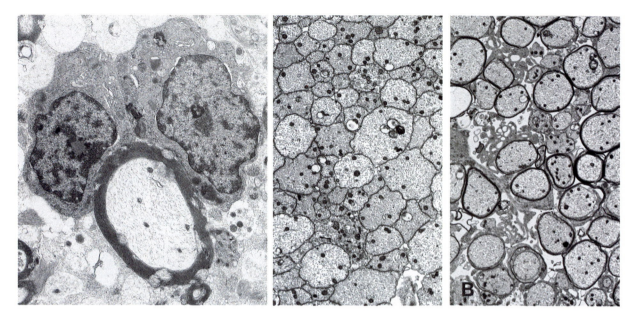

Figure 7.3 DEMYELINIZATION proceeds on several planes. Macrophages directly attack the myelin (*left*), presenting fragments of the protein on their surface for *T* cells to recognize. *T* cells attack from a distance by secreting cytokines, such as tumor necrosis factor. They also induce *B* cells to produce antibodies that destroy oligodendroglial cells, which normally repair myelin. The resulting demyelination (*center*) can be reversed by transplanting new oligodendroglial cells (*right*).

binds to HLA-DR2 and reduces the incidence of relapses in multiple sclerosis.

Another approach is to fight one of the *T* cells' principal chemical weapons: tumor necrosis factor. Feldmann and R. Tini Miani and their associates at the Kennedy Institute for Rheumatology in London and at Centocor Corporation have done so in a pilot trial. They produced a monoclonal antibody that binds with tumor necrosis factor and showed that it can clear that cytokine from the circulation. A single dose will suppress the autoimmune response for five to 10 weeks without damping the general immune response to infection. The potency of the treatment is matched only by its remarkable specificity.

Treatment with the antibody increased joint mobility and reduced the stiffness associated with rheumatoid arthritis. This strategy is also being contemplated to treat multiple sclerosis, in which tumor necrosis factor has been implicated as an agent of destruction at the scene of the disease in the white matter.

Yet another tactic is to distract the lymphocytes from their targets. Ted A. Yednock of Athena Neurosciences, Nati Karin of Stanford and I have pre-vented the development of EAE in rats in this fashion. We administered a monoclonal antibody directed to VLA-4, one of the adhesive protrusions from the *T* cell. A *T* cell that has been treated in this fashion cannot attach to matching receptors on the wall of the blood vessel. It therefore sails past its disembarkation point without even attempting to breach the blood-brain barrier. Not only were the animals protected from paralytic disease, their brains were also completely devoid of inflammation.

Such an approach is soon to be applied in multiple sclerosis. We have already humanized the anti-VLA-4 molecule—that is, we have substituted human components for those pieces that identify the molecule's murine origins. A similar approach was taken in an animal model of rheumatoid arthritis by Ko Okumura and his colleagues at the Juntendo University School of Medicine in Tokyo. They blocked lymphocyte migration to joints with an antibody to ICAM-1, a molecule that enables the cell to adhere to the blood vessel wall. Here, too, anti-ICAM-1 antibodies are now undergoing preclinical trials for use in human patients.

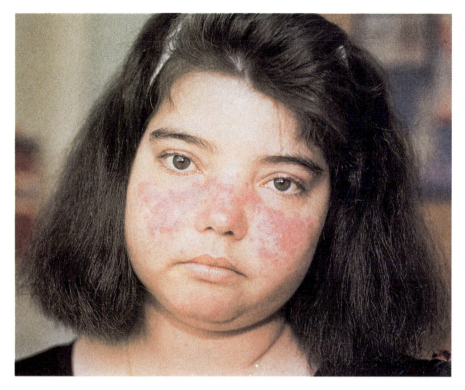

Figure 7.4 CHARACTERISTIC RASH over the cheekbones and forehead is diagnostic of systemic lupus erythemato- sus. The disease often begins in young adulthood and may eventually involve many organ systems.

An especially cunning approach has been undertaken by Caroline C. Whitacre of Ohio State University and Howard L. Weiner of Harvard University. They demonstrated that simply feeding myelin basic protein to animals with EAE can prevent or reverse paralysis. The mode of administering the protein matters, it seems, because the body is programmed to accept most proteins ingested as food and to attack most proteins that are presented directly to the tissues (as in a puncture wound or a subcutaneous injection). Such oral tolerance therapy, as it is called, appears to induce *T* cells that secrete cytokines—such as transforming growth factor β—that counteract the harmful effects of gamma-interferon and tumor necrosis factor.

Weiner recently conducted a small clinical trial in which he fed bovine myelin to multiple sclerosis patients and significantly reduced the number of relapses in the men, but not the women. Because the benefits were far more apparent in men than in women, the disparity perhaps can be linked to the effect estrogen has on the production of cytokines.

A more direct approach to the treatment of autoimmunity has aimed to remove specific subsets of *T* cells involved in the pathogenesis of disease. William J. Koopman and his colleagues at the University of Alabama at Birmingham have treated rheumatoid arthritis with a monoclonal anti-CD4 antibody. The antibody increased the mobility of the patients' joints considerably. This strategy is also being tested against multiple sclerosis by W. Ian McDonald and his co-workers at the National Hospital for Neurology and Neurosurgery in London.

The perfect treatment for autoimmunity would involve silencing or removing only the part of the immune system that is self-destructive, while leaving the rest intact to fight infection. This ideal may be more easily attained than researchers had originally thought because there is evidence that the *T* cells that cause autoimmune disease use a limited set of receptor molecules. The importance a single molecule may have was demonstrated most dramatically in EAE in 1988. In independent experiments, my colleagues and I at Stanford and Leroy E. Hood, then at the California Institute of Technology, and his co-workers showed that the T cells that induce paralysis in EAE all had the V-beta 8 gene, which encodes one of the components of the antigen receptor. We designed a monoclonal antibody directed to the product of that gene and showed that it reverses paralytic disease.

In the early 1980s Irun R. Cohen of the Weizmann Institute of Science had demonstrated that one could vaccinate individuals against their own rogue T cells and so prevent or even treat experimental autoimmune encephalomyelitis, experimental arthritis and experimental diabetes [see "The Self, the World and Autoimmunity," by Irun R. Cohen; SCIENTIFIC AMERICAN, April 1988].

Clinical trials with T cell vaccination have been initiated in multiple sclerosis and in rheumatoid arthritis. In 1989, in separate experiments, Offner-Vandenbark and Vandenbark and Steven W. Brostoff of Immune Response Corporation successfully treated EAE by vaccinating animals with a peptide from one of the T cell receptor molecules. Since then, Offner-Vandenbark and Vandenbark have tested the technique in a small number of multiple sclerosis patients, using a peptide found in a T cell receptor that reacts to myelin basic protein. Half of the patients exhibited an immune response to these pathogenic T cell receptors. Trials are now establishing whether this treatment alters the course of the disease.

As highly selective therapies for these diseases emerge, scientists will shift their focus to the repair of damaged tissues. Some such repair may be expected to proceed spontaneously, once the autoimmune response is interrupted. Moses Rodriguez and his colleagues at the Mayo Foundation have cited suggestive data from an animal model of multiple sclerosis. When the workers treated the animals by blocking the relevant T cells and HLA molecules, myelin was regenerated in the affected parts of the brain. More aggressive therapies may help speed such regeneration or induce it in cases where the damage is too profound to allow for self-repair. When Marc Noble and his associates at the Ludwig Institute for Cancer Research in London transplanted oligodendroglial cells into the brains of rodents with EAE, the grafts wrapped the ravaged regions with newly formed myelin.

This research may bear even richer fruits than anyone could have anticipated, for autoimmunity is turning out to be surprisingly widespread. It appears to complicate many diseases whose primary cause has nothing to do with immune response. In Duchenne's muscular dystrophy, for instance, a defective gene enfeebles a material crucial to the strength of muscle, weakening the person and finally leading to death from respiratory failure, usually in the patient's twenties. When the muscles were found to harbor T cells, immunosuppressive drugs were applied, prolonging the ability to walk by between three and five years.

Intriguing evidence suggests an even more momentous connection. Atherosclerosis, the arterial blockage that causes stroke and heart attack, may also involve autoimmunity. Among the signs are autoantibodies bound to fatty deposits in the arteries, histocompatibility proteins expressed in aberrant fashion, infiltration of macrophages and T cells secreting cytokines. These cytokines may induce the proliferation of smooth muscle and endothelial tissue that adds to the blockage. Should the connection prove real, therapies to suppress rogue T cells and their chemical messengers may one day reduce the severity of cardiovascular disease, the cause of half the deaths in the industrialized world.

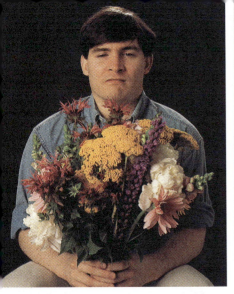
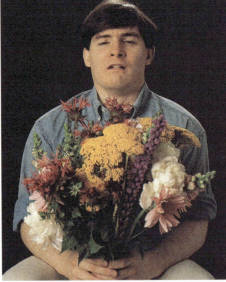
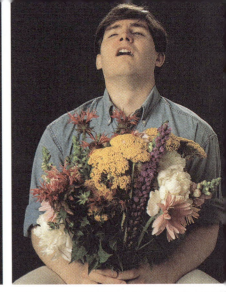
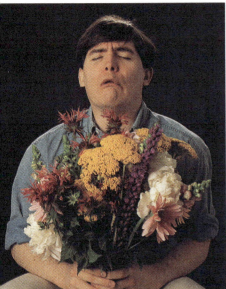
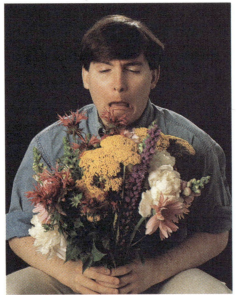
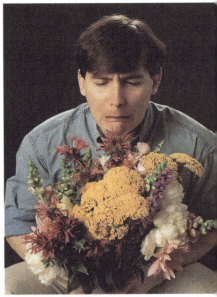
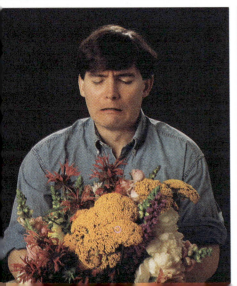
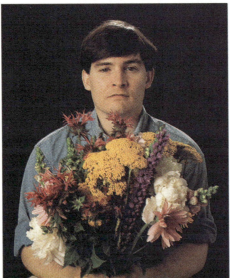
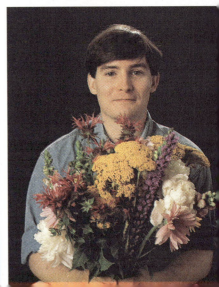

Allergy and the Immune System

In allergic individuals, parts of the immune system misdirect their power at innocuous substances, producing sometimes deadly symptoms.

· · ·

Lawrence M. Lichtenstein

The allergic response—in which certain components of the immune system react strongly to a normally inoffensive foreign substance—accounts for a good deal of the illness and medical expense in developed countries. Indeed, an estimated 20 percent or more of the U.S. population is allergic to something. The largest group suffers from allergic rhinitis (including hay fever) or asthma, sneezing (see Figure 8.1) or fighting for air after inhaling particular pollens or other ordinarily benign chemicals. Many children and some adults are allergic to foods. Others fall ill after receiving such medicines as penicillin. Still others endure untoward local or systemic reactions to bee stings. Occasionally, allergic attacks are fatal. Asthma alone accounted for an estimated \$3.6 billion in direct medical expenditures in 1990 and for nearly 1 percent of all health care costs.

To ease the financial, physiological and psychological burdens imposed by the wayward immune response, many researchers, including my colleagues and me at Johns Hopkins University, have long sought to expand existing therapeutic options. As part of this effort, we are attempting to uncover each step in the process by which exposure to an allergic trigger, or allergen, leads to symptoms. It is now clear that a number of the cellular and molecular interactions constituting the allergic response are often similar from person to person, regardless of differences in the substances to which the individuals react and the symptoms they exhibit. Many details of these exchanges remain to be deciphered, but recent discoveries are already generating exciting new ideas for prevention and control of allergic disorders.

Before addressing these discoveries, it seems worthwhile to examine the broader question of why natural selection has allowed allergy to become so widespread. An especially persuasive proposal derives from the observation that certain features of allergy occur in only one other circumstance: when the immune system attempts to eradicate parasites. For instance, in the response to both allergens and parasites, the body produces high quantities of molecules known as immunoglobulin E (IgE) antibodies. In contrast, when the immune system combats other invaders, notably bacteria, it relies on different classes of antibodies.

The hypothesis suggests that the allergic response initially evolved to help the body cope with parasites. People whose genetic endowment enabled them to mount an effective immune attack

Figure 8.1 SNEEZING triggered when an allergic individual inhales pollen results from a complex chain of molecular and cellular interactions in the nasal passages. Similar interactions underlie the symptoms evoked by other allergens.

against these organisms would have enjoyed a survival advantage, living longer than their counterparts who lacked such a defense mechanism. They would thus have produced more offspring, who in turn would have passed the helpful genes to their own, numerous children. In consequence, the parasite defense system became common in the human population. This defensive capability has remained useful wherever parasites are abundant. In people who no longer encounter these microbes, however, the immune system is now free to react—albeit counterproductively—to other substances, such as ragweed pollen.

In support of this thesis, epidemiologists find that allergic disease is less common in developing than in developed nations, where public health measures have eliminated most exposure to parasites. Yet animal studies designed to test the proposal have been inconclusive, and so the question of why allergy exists remains unsolved.

Understanding of the physiological basis of the allergic response rests on a more substantial collection of evidence. I can therefore offer a reasonably cohesive overview of current knowledge. We know, for instance, that different allergens evoke disparate symptoms in part because they engage with the immune system at separate sites in the body. In the upper airways the misdirected immune response yields sneezing and nasal congestion—in other words, allergic rhinitis. In the lower airways it can cause constriction and obstruction of the bronchi, thereby participating in the development of such asthmatic symptoms as wheezing. Likewise, immune activity in tissue of the gastrointestinal tract may at times cause nausea, abdominal cramps, diarrhea or vomiting.

Finally, if an allergen delivered via any route makes its way into the bloodstream, it can induce anaphylaxis—allergic reactions at sites distant from the port of entry into the blood. Severe anaphylactic reactions can disturb normal functioning throughout the body and may end in death.

Although the overt manifestations of the allergic response can vary, the response is universally set in motion by a silent process called sensitization (see boxed figure "Stages of an Allergic Reaction"). Sensitization may begin the first time an allergen, typically a protein, enters the body. In the airways or other tissues the allergy-inducing substance encounters scavenger cells, or macrophages. These cells engulf the foreign substance, chop it into

Stages of an Allergic Reaction

1. SENSITIZATION

The initial meeting of an allergen and the immune system yields no symptoms; rather it may prepare the body to react promptly to future encounters with the substance. The sensitization process begins when macrophages degrade the allergen and display the resulting fragments to *T* lymphocytes (*bottom left*). The steps that follow are somewhat obscure, but in a process involving secretion of interleukin-4 by *T* cells, *B* lymphocytes mature into plasma cells able to secrete allergen-specific molecules known as immunoglobulin E (IgE) antibodies. These antibodies attach to receptors on mast cells in tissue and on basophils circulating in blood.

2. ACTIVATION OF MAST CELLS

In later encounters between the allergen and the body, allergen molecules promptly bind to IgE antibodies on mast cells (*top left*). When one such molecule connects with two IgE molecules on the cell surface, it draws together the attached IgE receptors, thereby activating various enzymes (*green spheres*) in the cell membrane. Cascades involving tyrosine kinase enzymes, phospholipase C, protein kinase C and an influx of calcium ions (*black arrows*) induce chemical-laden granules to release their contents. These cascades appear to promote the synthesis and extrusion of cytokines (*brown arrows*). Other sequences of molecular interactions (*green arrows*) end in the secretion of such lipids as prostaglandins and leukotrienes. The chemicals released by mast cells are responsible for many allergic symptoms. The reaction pathways shown are but a sampling of those thought to occur; many are also only partly understood (*broken arrows*).

3. PROLONGED IMMUNE ACTIVITY

Chemicals emitted by active mast cells (*left*) and their neighbors in tissue may induce basophils, eosinophils and other cells flowing through blood vessels (*right*) to migrate into that tissue. The chemicals facilitate migration by promoting the expression and activity of adhesion molecules on the circulating cells and on vascular endothelial cells. The circulating cells then attach to the endothelial cells, roll along them and, eventually, cross between them into the surrounding matrix. These recruited cells secrete chemicals of their own (*orange speckles*), which can sustain immune activity and damage tissue.

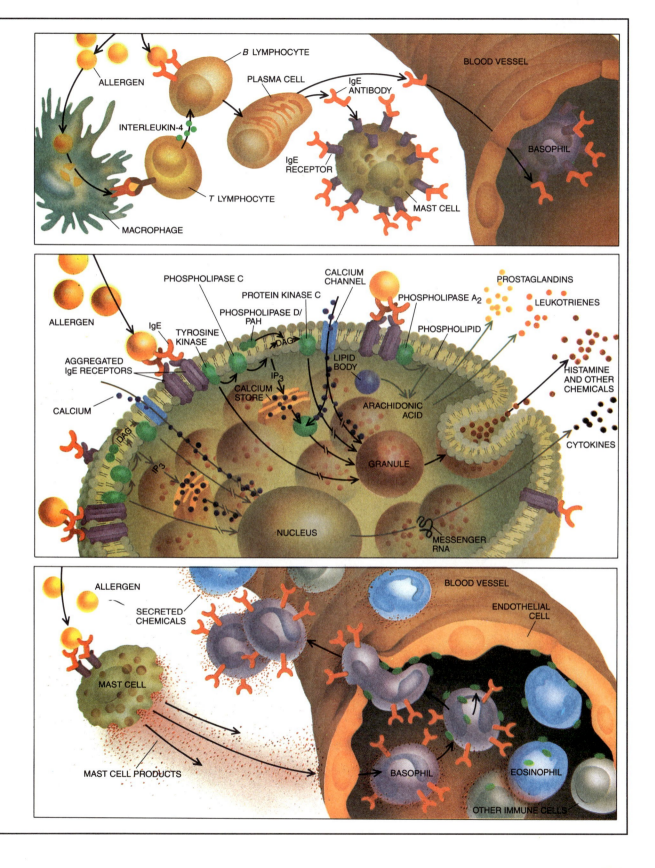

pieces and display the resulting fragments on the cell surface.

The sensitization process continues in the form of several incompletely understood interactions. In essence, however, leukocytes, or white blood cells, called helper *T* lymphocytes recognize certain of the displayed fragments and bind to them. Binding spurs the *T* cells to secrete interleukin-4 and other chemicals that prod neighboring *B* lymphocytes to mature into antibody-secreting plasma cells. At some point, the plasma cells switch from making so-called IgM antibodies to producing IgE antibodies. In common with other classes of antibodies, these molecules are Y-shaped; each "arm" is able to bind to one molecule of the allergen.

By the time the antibodies are made, days or weeks may have passed, and the allergen that elicited their production may be long gone. But the IgE molecules do not disappear. They attach by the "stem" of the Y to IgE receptors on two classes of immune system cells. One class consists of mast cells, which derive from bone marrow and reside in tissues (see Figure 8.2). Mast cells generally settle close to blood vessels and to the epithelium: the layer of epithelial and gland cells that covers the surfaces by which we make contact with the outer world. IgE antibodies also bind to basophils; these cells, too, derive from bone marrow, but they

differentiate into white cells that circulate in the bloodstream.

Once IgE antibody production begins, it apparently persists for months or, at times, many years. As a result, IgE antibodies perpetually occupy IgE receptors on mast cells and basophils, where they sit ready to react promptly to the next encounter with an allergen. Thus, even in a person who will later be revealed as allergic, the initial encounter evokes no symptoms; rather it primes the immune system to react to a subsequent exposure.

This later exposure initiates a more visible stage of the allergic response. Within seconds after an allergen meets human tissue, it binds to IgE antibodies on mast cells. When it engages at least two IgE molecules, it forms a bridge between them; this cross-linking, in turn, draws the attached IgE receptors close to one another. Such aggregation of receptors activates the cell. That is, it induces the cell to release potent chemicals that directly and indirectly generate allergic symptoms. (A number of triggers can independently elicit release of the same chemicals, but the resulting response typically is not classified as allergic if IgE antibodies are not involved.)

Among the released chemicals, mast cells produce two well-studied, symptom-causing groups referred to collectively as allergic mediators. One

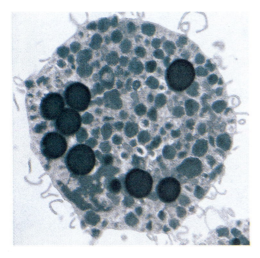
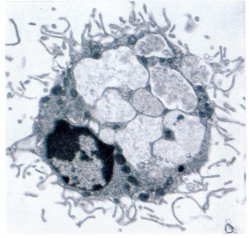

Figure 8.2 HUMAN MAST CELLS look quite different before (*left*) and after (*right*) activation. Activated cells retain very few granules (*small black spheres*) and display extensive alteration of the surface. The large spheres in the cell at the left are lipid bodies, which may participate in synthesizing the lipids secreted by stimulated mast cells. (Ann M. Dvorak of Harvard Medical School supplied the micrographs.)

set is synthesized in advance of antigen binding and is stored in microscopic granules. IgE cross-linking induces granules to fuse with the cell membrane and eject their contents.

Histamine, first described in 1911 by Sir Henry Dale of the Wellcome Physiological Research Laboratories in England, is perhaps the most infamous of these pre-formed mediators. It can stimulate the production of mucus from the epithelium, thereby contributing to congestion of airways. It can cause smooth muscles, which wrap like an elastic band around the bronchial airways and the intestines, to contract. Histamine can also dilate small blood vessels and increase their permeability, allowing fluid to leak into tissues. These vascular changes can give rise to redness and swelling. If the changes are widespread, they may contribute to a deadly condition termed hypotensive shock: a profound drop in blood pressure, accompanied by a dramatic reduction in the supply of oxygen to the heart and brain.

The second group of mediators, discovered decades later at the Karolinska Institute in Stockholm, consists of lipids (fats)—mainly prostaglandins and leukotrienes—that are synthesized after allergen molecules make contact with IgE antibodies on cells. Like histamine, both kinds of lipids cause constriction of the bronchial tubes and vascular dilatation; what is worse, their effects persist longer. Stimulated mast cells additionally extrude a variety of potentially toxic enzymes. Evidence suggests the cells release cytokines as well: small proteins that direct the activities of other immune system cells. Sometimes, virtually all the symptoms of an allergic attack seem to stem from the rapid release of mediators and other chemicals from mast cells. For example, swift activation of these cells is probably at fault in anaphylactic reactions or when a cat owner's hospitality is met with sneezes and tears by a visitor allergic to feline dander.

In most instances, though, the allergic reaction progresses to a third, often chronic, stage. At these times, it is thought that activated mast cells lure other immune system cells from the circulation into tissues. These attracted cells include basophils (which, like mast cells, contain granules) and granular white cells known as eosinophils. They also include *T* lymphocytes and monocytes (precursors of tissue macrophages). The presence of large numbers of basophils and eosinophils in an inflammatory lesion—tissue invaded by components of the immune system—constitutes another shared hallmark of allergy and parasitic infection. These cells are virtually absent at sites of bacterial invasion, where leukocytes known as neutrophils are more prominent.

The recruited cells secrete substances that can prolong and exacerbate the early symptoms and may injure local tissue. For example, basophils (which are activated in much the same way as mast cells) emit many of the pre-formed and lipid mediators also found in mast cells. Eosinophils release toxic proteins; one, major basic protein, can damage respiratory epithelial cells.

Current understanding of this third stage—often referred to as the late-phase reaction—derives from experiments done in my laboratory at Johns Hopkins University and elsewhere. In a standard technique, investigators study the effects of allergens by delivering them directly to the airways or into the skin of allergic volunteers. At the cellular level, the acute phase (mast cell activation in tissue) is followed hours later in many subjects by a late-phase inflammatory response: basophils and an army of other leukocytes invade the airways or skin, generating a new wave of symptoms. Varied data make me suspect that in the experimental situation, and probably in nature, basophils orchestrate much of the late response; the chemicals they secrete seem both to cause symptoms and to help sustain activity by the other cells.

Within minutes after a patient inhales an allergen, the cellular activities of the acute phase manifest themselves as sneezing and congestion or wheezing and shortness of breath. The symptoms disappear within an hour but return a few hours after that, paralleling the late-phase invasion of circulating cells into the epithelium. Similarly, delivery of allergens into the skin evokes an acute wheal-and-flare reaction (see Figure 8.3), or swelling and redness, followed later by prolonged return of the reaction. In the course of daily living, people do not necessarily experience delayed symptoms after an acute allergy attack. But ongoing exposure to allergens in sensitized individuals may result in persistent late-phase inflammation and in continuous or easily evoked symptoms.

Much of what I have just described has been established for some time. It is in the filling in of details, however, that new ideas for treatment arise. One area actively being studied focuses on an early part of the allergic response: regulation of

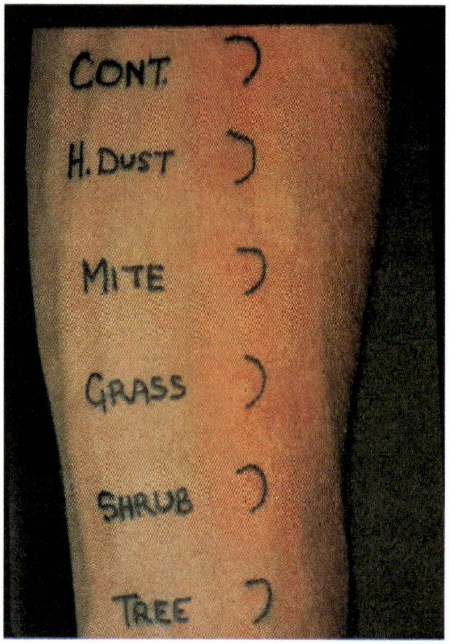

Figure 8.3 WHEAL-AND-FLARE REACTION—swelling and redness—indicates a person is allergic to a substance that has been injected into the skin. In this case, the reaction on the arm indicates the individual is allergic to grass.

IgE antibody synthesis. Why do allergic individuals generate abnormally high levels of IgE antibodies? (The concentrations of non-IgE antibodies in the blood typically vary little from person to person, whereas those of IgE antibodies can vary considerably. In allergic individuals, IgE levels remain much lower than those of other antibody classes, but they can be thousands of times higher than those in nonallergic people.)

Part of the explanation for the unusually high levels may rest with the nature of T cells active in allergic patients. Intriguing recent discoveries imply that the T cells in allergic lesions include two varieties—Th1 and Th2—and that the Th2 type predominates. It is also known that Th2 cells secrete interleukin-4 and interleukin-5 but not gamma-interferon, whereas Th1 cells secrete gamma-interferon and interleukin-2 but not interleukin-4 and interleukin-5. Interleukin-4 encourages B lymphocytes to make IgE antibodies rather than other types. Moreover, gamma-interferon retards such synthesis. These results suggest that an individual's mix of Th1 and Th2 cells determines whether B cells give rise to IgE molecules or other types of antibodies. Further, drugs able to interfere with the synthesis or activity of interleukin-4 might help reduce IgE levels and thus prevent allergic reactions.

Many workers, focusing on the effects rather than synthesis of IgE antibodies, are now attempting to trace the complex signal-transduction pathways in mast cells and basophils: the series of steps by which cross-linking of IgE molecules at the cell surface leads to the release of disease-inducing chemicals. In a critical breakthrough, the genes specifying the three types of protein that constitute the receptor for IgE antibodies have been cloned, providing important clues to the receptor's three-dimensional structure. As the precise functions of the receptor's subunits are discerned, specific blockade of their distinctive activities, and hence of mediator release, should be possible.

It is also clear that when an allergen binds to two or more IgE molecules and draws together the attached receptors, receptor aggregation switches on several separate biochemical cascades. Researchers have realized for a while that at least one cascade ending in the extrusion of mediators from granules depends on activity of the enzyme protein kinase C. They have found, too, that the enzyme phospholipase A2 is a central player in the secretion of leukotrienes and prostaglandins. More recent evidence indicates that various tyrosine kinases (enzymes that add phosphate groups to tyrosine amino acids on proteins) set off additional cascades that promote the disgorging of chemicals stowed in granules. Because many reaction pathways end in the same outcome—secretion of particular mediators and cytokines—therapies that block a single pathway may be incompletely successful on their own. The interruption of two or more pathways seems to be synergistic, however.

Compounds that inhibit enzymes involved in generating specific mediators are already in development. The prototypical therapeutic agent impedes activity of an enzyme called 5-lipoxygenase and in so doing retards production of several leukotrienes. Early trials of this inhibitor in asthmatic patients indicate that this approach will reduce inflammation.

Beyond signal transduction, we must explain how basophils, eosinophils and other white cells are recruited to sites where mast cells are active. The general consensus holds that stimulation of mast cells triggers the release of chemicals that penetrate into local, small blood vessels and increase expression of adhesion molecules on circulating leukocytes and on endothelial cells that line the interior of the vessels (see boxed figure "Mediators of Allergic Reaction"). The secreted chemi-

Mediators of Allergic Reactions

Molecules released from activated mast cells and basophils account for many allergic symptoms. This list includes a sampling of those chemicals and some of their effects, which can be redundant.

	CHEMICAL	ACTIVITY	SYMPTOMS
MEDIATORS FROM GRANULES	Histamine	Constricts bronchial airways	Wheezing; difficulty breathing
		Dilates blood vessels	Local redness at sites of allergen delivery; if dilatation is widespread, it can contribute to a lethal drop in blood pressure (shock)
		Increases permeability of small blood vessels	Swelling of local tissue; if change in permeability is widespread, it can contribute to shock
		Stimulates nerve endings	Itching and pain in skin
		Stimulates secretion of mucus in airways	Congestion of airways
	Platelet-activating factor	Constricts bronchial airways	*Same as for histamine*
		Dilates blood vessels	*Same as for histamine*
LIPID MEDIATORS	Leukotrienes	Constrict bronchial airways	*Same as for histamine*
		Increase permeability of small blood vessels	*Same as for histamine*
	Prostaglandin D	Constricts bronchial airways	*Same as for histamine*

cals include leukotrienes, platelet-activating factor and probably cytokines; the adhesion molecules have such names as integrins, selectins and immun-oglobulin adhesion molecules. Next, the leukocytes stick to the blood vessel wall and roll along it. They then migrate between endothelial cells and out into the surrounding tissue.

There the mixture of chemicals produced by diverse cell types controls their migration route, how far they travel and whether they will die or thrive. For instance, interleukin-3 and interleukin-5 (cytokines made by *T* cells) and GM-CSF (another cytokine, made by endothelial cells, macrophages and other cell types) facilitate the migration of eosinophils and basophils and may prolong their survival. A fourth cytokine, RANTES, made by *T* lymphocytes and other cells, seems to regulate migration by eosinophils.

Apparently, then, many different cells and molecules, not a single chemical, account for the presence of any given cell type in an allergic lesion. If the combinations of factors responsible for the accumulation of eosinophils and basophils in the allergic process can be clarified, this step, too, should become amenable to pharmaceutical control.

It is often useful to discuss allergy as if it were a single disease, but investigators are also giving attention to the best ways to diagnose and treat specific allergic conditions. Of these, allergic rhinitis is the most prevalent, affecting perhaps 15 percent of Americans.

This disorder takes two forms. People afflicted with one variant—hay fever—undergo symptoms seasonally; they may react to pollens of trees and grasses in the spring or to pollens of weeds in the fall. In the perennial variant, symptoms are more likely to be caused by indoor allergens, such as animal danders or the ubiquitous dust mite (see Figure 8.4). Allergic rhinitis is never fatal but may lead to complications, such as sinusitis, polyps or asthma. It is also a major nuisance and a cause of significant discomfort. Indeed, billions of dollars are spent every year to prevent and assuage the symptoms.

Physicians confirm the diagnosis by observing a wheal-and-flare reaction after tiny amounts of a suspected airborne allergen are injected into the skin. Antihistamines generally prove effective and are still the standard treatment. The newest versions of these drugs do not pass across the blood-brain barrier readily and so do not cause

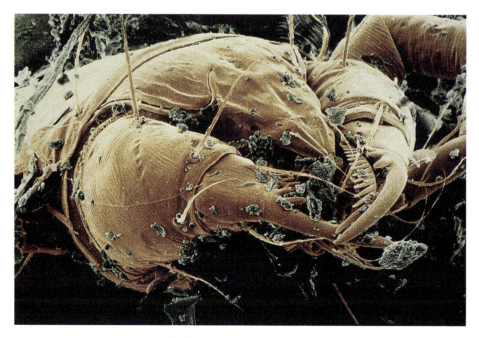

Figure 8.4 DUST MITE, invisible to the unaided eye, is a common cause of chronic allergic rhinitis. The allergic response is triggered by inhalation of the mite's feces.

drowsiness. When inflammation is severe and antihistamines are ineffective, compounds more commonly prescribed to alleviate the chronic inflammation of asthma (that is, inhaled corticosteroids) are often helpful. I anticipate that experimental drugs now being tested on asthmatics, which I shall discuss later, could offer added alternatives for allergic rhinitis sufferers.

For severe cases, immunotherapy (also called allergy shots or desensitization), which was introduced in 1911, may provide relief. Physicians inject patients with increasing doses of the allergens to which they are sensitive. I wish I could describe how immunotherapy confers resistance to an allergen, but no one has put forward a definitive explanation. Nevertheless, controlled studies by A. William Frankland of St. Mary's Hospital in London and Francis C. Lowell of Harvard University in the 1950s demonstrated that immunotherapy for grass and ragweed sensitivity can ameliorate allergic rhinitis and asthma. My colleagues and I later confirmed this observation, and others demonstrated that allergens produced by dust mites can be useful as well. In all cases, however, the dosage is critical; too little allergen provides no protection. Moreover, protection is rarely complete.

Asthma is much more serious than allergic rhinitis and is sometimes lethal. Roughly 5 to 10 percent of children have the condition, about a third of whom may display no symptoms after adolescence. Conversely, another 5 to 10 percent of people acquire asthma in adulthood; it may arise at any time, even in one's eighties.

As is true of allergic rhinitis, asthma is generally divided into two types. In the extrinsic form, an offending allergen can be identified; in the intrinsic form, symptoms cannot be traced to a substance capable of inciting production of IgE antibodies. Actually, though, the defining features of asthma can probably result from any of at least half a dozen different disease processes, some of which may involve IgE-mediated activity, and some of which may not.

One hallmark of the disease is so-called twitchy airways. Compared with the bronchi of nonasthmatics, those of asthmatics contract in response to much lower doses of bronchoconstrictors (such as histamine or methacholine) or of noxious substances (such as ozone or tobacco smoke). In asthmatics, exercise and cold, dry air can bring on symptoms as well.

Asthmatics may also evince chronic but potentially reversible partial obstruction of their lower airways. Much of the obstruction is thought to arise from inflammatory processes resembling those seen in the late-phase response produced in the laboratory. Evidently, chemicals released from mast cells and infiltrating basophils combine with toxic eosinophil proteins to promote mucus production, as well as to damage tissue, thicken airway walls and, perhaps, increase bronchial hyperreactivity. When an allergen comes along, the resulting constriction of the airways can then close the already partially occluded passages.

Bronchodilators are the most commonly used drugs for asthma; they relieve the symptoms generated by histamine and other bronchoconstrictors soon after exposure to an allergen. Yet these drugs probably do not affect the underlying inflammation. Further, overuse of bronchodilators may cause "rebound" constriction and actually decrease airflow. Prevailing wisdom favors ongoing treatment of the inflammatory process in addition to separate treatment of acute episodes.

The approved anti-inflammatory agents include corticosteroids and nonsteroidal drugs. Of these, the steroids are the most potent. Until about a decade ago, patients generally took the steroids orally, and the side effects (such as weight gain, osteoporosis and ulcers) posed a major problem. More recently many studies have shown that the inhaled, or topically administered, versions can achieve good control without producing significant unwelcome effects. On the other hand, inhaled steroids may not attain full effectiveness in people who undergo very frequent asthmatic attacks or who have perpetual breathing difficulties.

This last problem has spurred a search for anti-inflammatory agents that are more potent than corticosteroids but also relatively nontoxic. Two of the more exciting classes of drug candidates aim to block the activity of inflammatory cytokines and the adhesion molecules that facilitate migration of immune system cells from the blood into tissue. In theory, such products should ameliorate not only asthma but many allergic disorders, including some that are not now amenable to treatment (such as chronic skin allergies). These drugs have not yet entered clinical trials for the treatment of asthma, but preliminary studies in humans and other primates are encouraging.

Research into experimental therapies for asthma does not end there. In addition to developing drugs that should block enzymes involved in signal transduction, pharmaceutical houses are devising new products that interfere with the activity of mediators made by mast cells and basophils. For instance, several companies are well into clinical trials of substances that block the functioning of leukotrienes. The drugs reduce symptoms and may work even better when combined with antihistamines. (Antihistamines by themselves do not have much effect in asthmatics, presumably because inflammatory cells secrete large amounts of leukotrienes and other redundant mediators.)

Investigators also continue to explore the value of immunotherapy for asthmatics. This treatment is offered more often by allergists than pulmonary specialists. When such a disparity exists in medicine, it means that the treatment is not dramatically or completely effective in most patients. A recent study conducted by the National Institutes of Health showed that ragweed immunotherapy could benefit asthmatics, but the effect was modest.

Sadly, the incidence of asthma and the number of deaths it causes surged by more than 60 percent in the 1980s. The reasons for the rises are mysterious, as is the explanation for why Americans of African descent are three times more likely than those of European descent to die from the disease. Hypotheses to explain the overall mortality figures range from overuse or ineffectual use of bronchodilators to an increase in environmental pollutants and allergens. In the African-American population, poor access to care may also be at fault.

Just as asthma can be deadly, so too can anaphylaxis, which is frightening for both the patient and the physician treating it. It was first described in 2641 B.C.: a tablet describes the death of the Egyptian king Menes after an insect sting. In the U.S. today, millions of anaphylactic reactions probably occur every year, although deaths apparently number in the hundreds.

The symptoms, which can vary, result from an acute, explosive release of chemicals from mast cells (see boxed figure "After a Sting"). This explosion typically elicits one or more symptoms within minutes, and it can kill promptly. Shock is a major cause of death. People can also perish if the vocal cords swell (as a result of blood fluid leaking into tissues) and close off the trachea. This disturbance is one of the few that is readily corrected, by tracheotomy. Making a hole in the trachea just below the "Adam's apple"—be it with a scalpel or even a table knife or the tip of a fountain pen—can be lifesaving. Other possible manifestations of mast cell activity include asthmalike constriction of the lower airways. Skin eruptions and itching are particularly common, whereas gastrointestinal disturbances occur rarely.

Interestingly, in individuals who have undergone repeated episodes of anaphylaxis, the particular set of symptoms suffered almost always reproduces itself exactly. These symptoms may be preceded by an aura, in which the patient may have a feeling of impending doom or, strangely, a feeling of great calm or peace. Whether severe anaphylaxis is occurring for the first time or the fifteenth, it is an emergency. Hence, treatment must focus on correcting the most serious symptoms. Usually this strategy includes injection of epinephrine (adrenaline), which inhibits mediator release, opens airways and combats dilatation of blood vessels. Naturally, the best treatment is avoidance. In the case of bee stings, this strategy is often impossible, and so immunization with the venom of the offending insect is used to prevent reactions.

Bee-sting immunotherapy has an instructive history that underscores the importance of well-designed clinical trials of new therapies. Back in 1930, in the first volume of *Journal of Allergy*, Robert L. Benson and Herman Semenov of the University of Oregon described a single case of a beekeeper who suffered an anaphylactic reaction to a sting. Searching for the allergens that might be delivered as a preventive, they performed skin tests on this patient with bee venom (later identified as the true allergen) and with ground-up whole bees. They found that the patient responded equally to both these preparations. They therefore concluded that allergic patients could be helped with whole-body extracts, which were significantly less difficult and expensive to produce than venom.

Unfortunately, they failed to realize that beekeepers would test positive to both venom and body parts of bees because they continually inhale the constituents of the dead insects and consequently become sensitive to those constituents. Allergic individuals in the general population encounter bees less often and do not become so sensitized.

Based on this single case report, physicians "immunized" allergic patients with whole-body

After a Sting

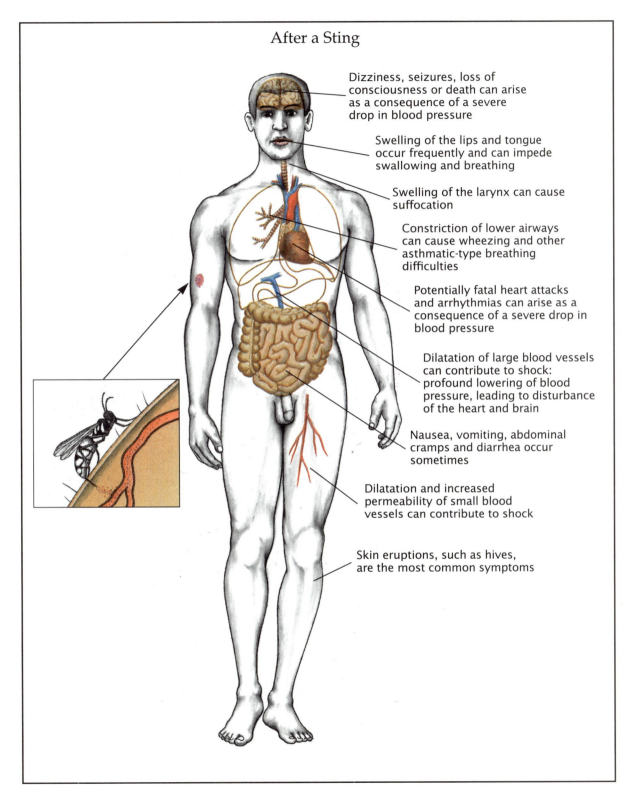

Dizziness, seizures, loss of consciousness or death can arise as a consequence of a severe drop in blood pressure

Swelling of the lips and tongue occur frequently and can impede swallowing and breathing

Swelling of the larynx can cause suffocation

Constriction of lower airways can cause wheezing and other asthmatic-type breathing difficulties

Potentially fatal heart attacks and arrhythmias can arise as a consequence of a severe drop in blood pressure

Dilatation of large blood vessels can contribute to shock: profound lowering of blood pressure, leading to disturbance of the heart and brain

Nausea, vomiting, abdominal cramps and diarrhea occur sometimes

Dilatation and increased permeability of small blood vessels can contribute to shock

Skin eruptions, such as hives, are the most common symptoms

extracts of bees and yellow jackets for the next half century, until my colleagues and I did a controlled study comparing the preventive value of a placebo, a whole-body extract and venom. We found that the whole-body extract did not differ in effectiveness from the placebo; in contrast, the venom was uniformly successful at forestalling bee-sting anaphylaxis. Thus, because of the lack of a controlled study, physicians treated their patients for years with a totally worthless material. Today only venom is administered.

Food allergies, which can cause local or systemic reactions, deserve special mention because of widespread misunderstandings about them. These allergies are not uncommon in children. In definitive studies, my colleague Hugh A. Sampson has demonstrated that affected youngsters usually are sensitive to proteins in milk, nuts or eggs. The symptoms, typically skin rashes, can be fairly subtle in children. To be sure of the diagnosis, at Johns Hopkins we perform a standard skin test. If that result is positive, we do a double-blind food-challenge test: on one day a capsule of an allergen or a placebo is fed to a child, and on another day the alternate choice is given. At the time of the feeding, neither the patient, the parent nor the physician knows whether a food or a placebo is being administered.

In adults the cause-and-effect relation between a food and symptoms is usually obvious because dramatic symptoms arise promptly. Most often, an individual will acquire hives (urticaria) or suffer a more serious anaphylactic reaction within minutes after eating shellfish or nuts. Hence, suspected allergy can be confirmed with a simple skin test. Probably dozens of people die every year because nuts or egg proteins unexpectedly show up in packaged or other foods.

Food allergies in adults are uncommon, affecting only 1 to 2 percent of the population. Yet about 25 percent of Americans believe they are allergic to some food and that this sensitivity engenders vague disturbances such as depression, fatigue or extreme irritability. I am perturbed by this phenomenon because there are doctors who minister to these patients, using completely unreliable tests to diagnose food sensitivity. I estimate that

hundreds of millions of dollars are thus wasted on useless tests and treatments every year.

These are not the most worrisome doctors. One group, self-described clinical ecologists, diagnose patients as being "sensitive" to their environment, such as to minor contaminants in water, food or air, even though these contaminants cannot, in fact, induce allergic responses. As before, these practitioners typically diagnose by unproved techniques; each method that has been examined in rigorous trials has been found wanting. Yet the clinical ecologists and their patients are highly outspoken, and so I fear that already limited federal research dollars will be alloted to the study of this so-called allergy to the environment.

Finally, many questionable types of immunotherapy are offered. For instance, those who employ the Rinkel technique inject tiny, homeopathic doses of allergens. Years ago several of my colleagues collaborated with advocates of the Rinkel approach to plan a careful study of their method. As would be expected from research demonstrating the need for relatively high doses, this study failed to prove any efficacy. In another odd practice, small amounts of a potentially offending inhaled allergen are placed under the tongue as a form of "desensitization." There is no evidence that this procedure works.

Those of us conducting research by the standard scientific method can feel heartened by the extent of progress that has been achieved to date. Even so, gaps remain. We need to understand the mechanisms of signal transduction in more detail, so that we can develop drugs to block the release of mediators and their relatives from immune cells. It is important to determine precisely which circulating cells are involved in causing allergic diseases and to discern exactly how they are drawn into inflammatory lesions. And we need to understand which of the many, redundant cellular secretions most contribute to distressing symptoms, so that we can develop effective antagonists. I am confident that the tools being honed by investigators in the pharmaceutical and biotechnology industries and in academia will help resolve these issues to a significant extent within the next few years.

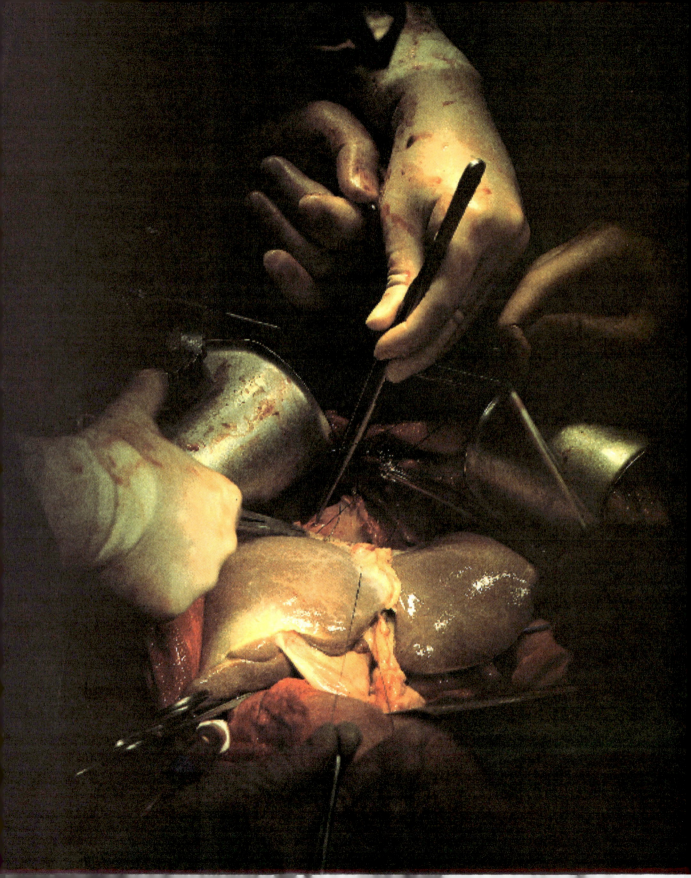

The Immune System as a Therapeutic Agent

New technologies and insights into the molecular underpinnings of the immune system provide the basis for novel approaches to vaccines and other therapies.

• • •

Hans Wigzell

The immune system is an alchemist's dream. Its multifaceted methods of attacking such intruders as bacteria or viruses offer researchers an abundance of compounds and molecular strategies that can extend the scope of medical intervention. Using our knowledge of the immune system, we can strengthen its response to a given antigen, direct it to combat an overlooked foe or, in cases of organ rejection, forestall misguided attacks (see Figure 9.1). When successful, these attempts give rise to a kind of gold in therapies to prevent and to treat disease.

Efforts are currently under way to improve existing vaccines, to make them more specific and to eliminate any adverse reactions that may accompany immunization. These refinements and a more thorough understanding of certain illnesses have suggested innovative means of limiting immune system responses in cases of allergy, autoimmunity and organ rejection by pinpointing and blocking the action of specific molecules. In contrast, other therapies are being crafted to increase attacks on cancer and AIDS. Perhaps most exciting

is the creative use of components of the immune system as biological mimics and as enzymes that can help in the treatment of disease.

In general, there are two approaches to harnessing the immune system therapeutically. Not surprisingly, these approaches reflect two aspects of immunologic function. Certain reactions of the immune system are antigen-specific, that is, selected T cells or antibodies respond to a precise target: a foreign organism or entity. The T cell form of action is called cell-mediated; the antibody response is termed humoral.

The second form of immune system reaction is not antigen-specific. This type of response entails the actions of compounds known as cytokines, which resemble hormones, or those of antibacterial peptides. Such molecules can destroy bacterial cell walls, prevent viruses from replicating or interfere with the biochemistry of pathogens in a number of other manners.

Therapeutic uses of the antigen-specific strategy are familiar because they include one of medicine's most potent defenses: vaccines against infectious diseases. The key to vaccines lies in the immune system's remarkable memory. Not only can it recognize and destroy nearly any intruder, the immune system also can remember for decades most of its previous skirmishes. Thus, when a person is given a weakened dose of an infectious agent such as the virus that causes polio (see

Figure 9.1 LIVER TRANSPLANT can cause the recipient's immune system to reject the donor organ after surgery. Recent discoveries in immunology are pointing toward ways in which the system can be safely manipulated to thwart its own efforts to attack such grafts.

Figure 9.2), his or her body responds by making antibodies and *T* cells that ultimately eliminate the virus. Once the organism has been obliterated, the responsible antibodies and *T* cells remain on the alert and protect the immunized individual against any later, and perhaps more virulent, encounters with the same organism.

Vaccinations of various kinds have been used for hundreds of years. Pliny the Elder thought the livers of mad dogs held a cure for rabies. And for centuries, Asian physicians took dried crusts from the lesions of smallpox patients and gave them to children to scratch into their skin or to inhale nasally. Many children became immunized, but some developed smallpox. It was not until 1796 that British physician Edward Jenner used a related virus, cowpox, to immunize people against smallpox effectively and safely.

At the turn of this century, techniques to make vaccines became somewhat more precise. Researchers grew microbes in laboratories and administered small doses of the killed or attenuated organisms as vaccines. The improvements, however, did not always ensure the purity of the product: disease sometimes resulted, and reactions to vaccines were not uncommon. After this advance, vaccine research proceeded at a painstakingly slow pace (see boxed figure "Events in the History of Vaccine Development").

Developments in the past decade have revived such investigations. Using molecular techniques, scientists can now rapidly locate the genetic component of a microorganism that gives rise to an illness. They can isolate the protein, or series of proteins, arising from these genes, manufacture it in pure form and in great quantity and then vaccinate people with the specific element rather than with the entire organism (see Figure 9.3). Furthermore, if any proteins in a potential vaccine are found to be harmful, they can now be easily deleted or modified.

Specificity increases a vaccine's effectiveness. Monoclonal antibodies can be used to discover the neutralizing determinant, or vulnerable portion, of a bacterium or virus. A large majority of the antibodies that the body produces to conquer an organism—say, an influenza virus—are ineffectual because they target proteins that do not allow them to eradicate the organism. But the remaining

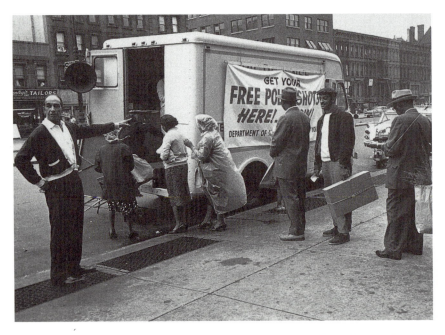

Figure 9.2 HARLEM RESIDENTS wait in line to receive a poliomyelitis vaccine at a mobile clinic in 1959. The unit was part of a health department drive to vaccinate everyone in New York City. Now that smallpox has been wiped out, World Health Organization officials have targeted the polio virus for eradication.

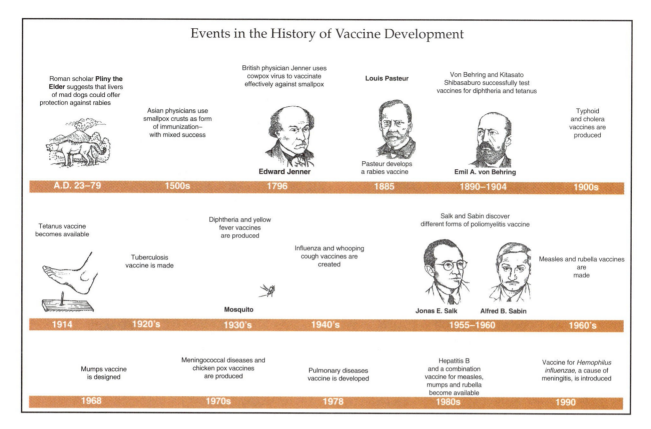

Events in the History of Vaccine Development

Roman scholar **Pliny the Elder** suggests that livers of mad dogs could offer protection against rabies

Asian physicians use smallpox crusts as form of immunization– with mixed success

British physician Jenner uses cowpox virus to vaccinate effectively against smallpox

Edward Jenner

Louis Pasteur

Pasteur develops a rabies vaccine

Von Behring and Kitasato Shibasaburo successfully test vaccines for diphtheria and tetanus

Emil A. von Behring

Typhoid and cholera vaccines are produced

| A.D. 23–79 | 1500s | 1796 | 1885 | 1890–1904 | 1900s |

Tetanus vaccine becomes available

Tuberculosis vaccine is made

Diphtheria and yellow fever vaccines are produced

Influenza and whooping cough vaccines are created

Mosquito

Salk and Sabin discover different forms of poliomyelitis vaccine

Jonas E. Salk **Alfred B. Sabin**

Measles and rubella vaccines are made

| 1914 | 1920's | 1930's | 1940's | 1955–1960 | 1960's |

Mumps vaccine is designed

Meningococcal diseases and chicken pox vaccines are produced

Pulmonary diseases vaccine is developed

Hepatitis B and a combination vaccine for measles, mumps and rubella become available

Vaccine for *Hemophilus influenzae*, a cause of meningitis, is introduced

| 1968 | 1970s | 1978 | 1980s | 1990 |

minority of antibodies are focused on a weakness in the viral defenses. Therefore, if a person receives a vaccine composed of the protein or proteins that make up the neutralizing site, his or her antibody production for that portion of the virus will increase, and disease will be staved off.

Such advances in vaccine design have been accompanied by more effective ways to administer immunizations. For instance, killer, or cytotoxic, *T* cells cannot attack an antigen unless it has been taken inside a cell and presented on a surface compound called the major histocompatibility complex (MHC). In the past, ensuring this absorption and subsequent correct presentation required that the vaccine be made of live organism or virus, a sometimes dangerous proposition.

New adjuvants (substances used in the preparation of vaccines) can circumvent this problem because they can ensure that an antigen will be "seen" by the correct immune system cell (see Figure 9.4). Researchers can insert an antigen into liposomes, or tiny capsules made of fatty molecules. Once the liposomes are in the body, macrophages devour them. Like waiters bringing dinner to ravenous diners, the macrophages and other immune system cells that have consumed the antigen-laden liposomes find themselves surrounded by *T* cells.

Another fascinating way of obtaining a killer *T* cell response entails injecting DNA that encodes a foreign protein into skeletal muscle. Although this serendipitous finding is not entirely understood, it seems that muscle cells, which are much larger than most body cells, can serve as factories where antigens are produced, processed and presented on the MHC molecules. The muscle cells make the foreign protein from the injected DNA and then offer it up as antigen that is recognizable to the *T* cells. Although there is an autoimmune response against the muscle cells, it appears to be negligible.

Despite these improvements in vaccines, many microorganisms maintain their capacity to outwit the immune system. Elusive quarry, including the malaria parasite, continuously alters its appearance as it rescrambles its genetic systems. Although a more complete understanding of the

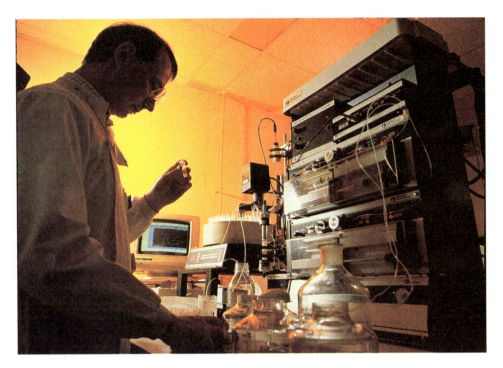

Figure 9.3 **LABORATORY TECHNOLOGY** has advanced dramatically in the past decade, thereby permitting the development of more selective and sophisticated vaccines. In this photograph, a researcher uses automated, computer-controlled equipment to produce monoclonal antibodies.

structure of these organisms or parasites will improve vaccine design, pathogens will always exist that are capable of resisting immunization.

The vaccines that I have just described are prophylactic; they are given before contact with a disease-causing organism. Vaccines that may serve as remedies have also been developed and have, like their cousins, benefited from the recent advances in molecular biology. Immunotherapy for patients who have allergies to pollen or to animal proteins, for instance, is undergoing a transformation. Traditional treatment of this problem involves the repeated administration of an allergen, say, cat hair, in highly dilute, gradually increasing concentrations. Such classical therapy can reduce a person's sensitivity to the allergen, but it works in only some patients, and its methods of action are constantly debated.

A more sophisticated alternative to vaccine therapy would attempt to disarm the antibodies involved in the reaction. The form of immediate allergy described above is usually caused by the overproduction of antibodies, or immunoglobulins, belonging to a class called IgE. Thus, a logical treatment would be to suppress IgE and IgE-related reactions.

It is known that two chemical messengers, interleukin-4 and interleukin-5, produced by T cells augment the production of IgE. Because many allergy-inducing organisms have an unusual ability to induce the formation of these compounds, vaccines could be designed to block interleukin-4 and interleukin-5. The potential success of this approach has been suggested in laboratory experiments on mice: rodents unable to produce interleukin-4 are also unable to make IgE. Another chemical messenger, gamma-interferon, brings about the production of molecules that inhibit the formation of interleukin-4 and interleukin-5. Therefore, vaccines developed to treat IgE-dependent allergies could include an agent that would lead to the production of gamma-interferon.

Curbing immune response is also the secret to preventing organ transplant rejections and to treating autoimmune disorders. The goal in transplan-

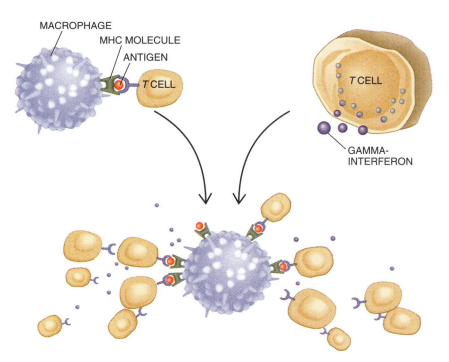

Figure 9.4 CHEMICAL MESSENGERS produced by the immune system, such as gamma-interferon (*small purple spheres at top right*), can be used to increase attacks on an antigen. Before an antigen can be "seen" by T cells, it must be processed by a macrophage and presented on a major **histocompatibility complex (MHC) molecule (*top left*). Gamma-interferon amplifies this process (*bottom*) by causing macrophages to display more antigen, thereby enhancing T cell activity.**

tation is to create specific tolerance in the recipient toward the antigens from the donor or, in the case of a bone marrow graft, to deter the lymphocytes produced in the donor marrow from attacking the recipient. We know this option is within reach in humans because nonidentical twins, who shared blood circulation during pregnancy, can accept tissue grafted from each other.

A spectacular means to achieve tolerance would be to harness an autoimmune response. The recipient's immune system could be used to identify and then wipe out T cells carrying receptors for the transplanted antigens. It has indeed been possible to induce autoimmunity against T cells with a specific antigen-binding capacity. I have been involved in several experiments in which rats from strain A were injected with T cells that sought the antigens from the tissue of rats from strain B.

We found that in a minority of animals the vaccination brought about lifelong specific tolerance against the *B* antigens, without complications. These exciting experiments have, however, been frustrating because it has proved impossible to make these autoimmune systems produce specific tolerance in a reproducible manner. Yet the fact that the experiments resulted in a low but specific number of animals becoming functionally tolerant illustrates the biological validity of the concept.

The most successful immune intervention for transplantation directs monoclonal antibodies against the cell-mediated part of the immune system. In fact, the first monoclonal antibody to be registered as a drug is targeted against the constant part of the antigen-binding receptor on T lymphocytes that are causing the rejection of a kidney transplant. (The constant portion remains the same in all T cells; the variable-gene portion changes, allowing antigenic specificity.) Unfortunately, although the drug reduces the rejection of the kidney, it has a major disadvantage because it blocks all T cell function.

Monoclonal antibodies with more selective immunosuppressive activity are being designed. Some are directed against CD4 or CD8 molecules of the *T* cells that bind with antigens, others against adhesion molecules on the *T* cell surface and still others against receptors for interleukins. Reportedly, several of these antibodies have been shown to be beneficial when used in preliminary trials in patients.

In addition to blocking immune system attacks on foreign antigens, vaccines have the potential to thwart attacks on the self. The causes of many autoimmune diseases—including rheumatoid arthritis, in which *T* cells attack joints, insulin-dependent diabetes, in which *T* cells attack insulin-making pancreatic cells, and multiple sclerosis, in which *T* cells attack the fatty sheaths around nerve cells—have been generally unknown. Animal models suggest that immunization with self-components can induce the autoimmune disease. For example, an injection of rat collagen can give rise to a rheumatoid arthritis–like disorder in the same animal. But until recently, it was unclear whether these models reflected what occurs in humans (see Chapter 7, "Autoimmune Disease," by Lawrence Steinman).

Regardless of etiology, enough is known about autoimmune disorders to permit vaccine research. The antigen-specific therapy for autoimmune disease has only two possible targets: the disease-inducing agent, or antigen, and the antigen-specific lymphocytes, or *T* cells, that are attacking the tissue. In the case of human autoimmune disease, the former are still not known. So one major strategy has been to eliminate selectively the *T* lymphocytes in the affected tissue. (Most autoimmune diseases are cell-mediated.)

The tactic is essentially to use autoimmunity to combat autoimmunity. When immunologists examine the local *T* cell populations causing a disease, they often find an enormous enrichment of *T* cells that recognize a certain antigen at the site of the illness. For example, my colleagues and I have seen that for an autoimmune lung disorder called sarcoidosis, 100 percent of the patients of a similar genetic background have an unusually large number of *T* cells with a characteristic receptor in their lungs.

In animal experiments, several groups have been able to immunize against variable-gene products that give rise to an identifiable receptor. In this way, one can block the activity of *T* cells having that particular antigen-binding receptor. After such immunizations, researchers have observed reduced numbers of *T* cells expressing the relevant variable-gene marker in addition to lowered immune function in cells that did express this marker. Immunization also resulted in protection against other autoimmune diseases that are characterized by *T* cells carrying this same receptor. Several teams have recently vaccinated patients with human variable-gene products. It will soon be known whether such immunizations result in an autoimmune attack against the relevant *T* lymphocytes and, if so, whether this finding has clinical applications.

In cases of autoimmunity, graft rejection and allergy, the immune system reaction needs to be scaled down and redirected. The opposite is true for AIDS and for cancer: the immune system attack needs to be scaled up. The desperate situation brought about by the human immunodeficiency virus (HIV), which causes AIDS, has prompted attempts to develop therapeutic vaccines, in addition to the ongoing efforts to design preventive vaccines. These experimental forays have not yielded any clinical benefits, but they have suggested intriguing avenues for research (see Figure 9.5).

One attempt involves isolating envelope proteins, called gp120 or gp160 (a combination of gp120 and gp41), from HIV. The protein is given to HIV-infected individuals in whom symptoms have not developed. As initially shown at the Walter Reed Army Institute of Research and confirmed by my colleagues at the Karolinska Institute, this procedure can generate an enhanced immune response against HIV. The reaction includes increased titers of antibodies that neutralize the envelope protein and other HIV variants. Normally, levels of CD4 *T* cells, which bind to HIV, drop in infected patients. Although this observation needs to be confirmed, there have been at least two reports that CD4 *T* cell decline is curbed following vaccination with the gp160 protein.

A second interesting candidate for a therapeutic HIV vaccine is based on autoimmunity. In a series of experiments, Norman L. Letvin and his group at Harvard University injected macaque monkeys with recombinant CD4 molecules in order to block infection. They found that the animals made antibodies against CD4. These antibodies appear to have no effect on normal CD4 *T* cell function, yet they inhibit HIV and SIV, the green monkey virus usually described as simian immunodeficiency

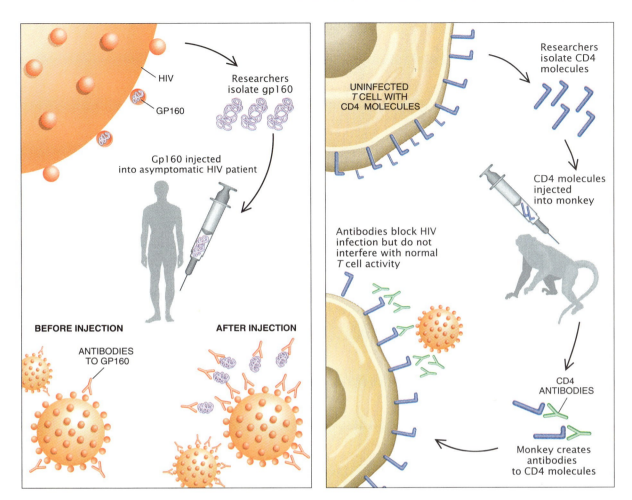

Figure 9.5 THERAPEUTIC AIDS VACCINES of two varieties are currently being tested. The first form (*left*) entails isolating a protein, called gp160 (which is composed of gp120 and gp41), from the human immunodeficiency virus (HIV). Gp160 is injected into an HIV-infected patient, causing the individual to make antibodies to the circulating protein and thereby increasing the number of antibodies available to attack the whole virus. The second type of vaccine (*right*) involves taking CD4 mol-ecules from *T* cells and injecting them into a macaque monkey. The animal responds by producing antibodies to the CD4 molecules; these antibodies bind to the CD4 molecules and prevent the virus from entering the *T* cells.

virus, from replication in vitro. Ostensibly, the antibodies work because they disturb the viral binding site on the cells and thereby prevent the virus from binding and entering the CD4 *T* cells. If the virus cannot gain entry, it cannot destroy the cells. Furthermore, immunization with recombinant CD4 molecules in SIV-infected monkeys caused a reduction or a disappearance of virus from the blood for up to four months.

The frequent appearance of normally rare cancers, including Kaposi's sarcoma, in AIDS patients has suggested to some researchers that the immune system is able to combat such tumors—although the role of the immune system in cancer suppression is hotly debated. Nevertheless, this possibility, coupled with observations that the immune system can sometimes overcome common cancers, forms the basis of some immunotherapeutic efforts to treat cancer.

Augmenting the early immune response to a tumor is pivotal. If the immune system could recognize and attack tumor-associated antigens before a tumor reached a critical size, the chances to wipe out the disease would be greatly enhanced [see "Teaching the Immune System to Fight Cancer," by Thierry Boon; SCIENTIFIC AMERICAN, March 1993]. This kind of early immune intervention is particularly promising for cancers in which viruses are implicated. These tumors exhibit tumor-associated antigens that are encoded by viral genes. When normal animal cells are injected with one of these viral genes, T lymphocytes are able to kill all cells expressing the antigen protein. In mouse tumors, similar vaccines administered after viral infection block the appearance of tumors.

In other cancers, tumor-associated molecules that serve as antigens may be caused by mutations in genes. These genes—oncogenes or suppressor genes for the oncogenes—are involved in cellular proliferation. Such mutations create new peptides, or antigens, against which T cells may respond. Intensive research is now under way to explore whether this latter strategy can be used to produce vaccines capable of inducing a therapeutic immune response against already established tumors.

In general, killer T cells are more destructive than antibodies. Unfortunately, most T cells are ineffective against many tumor-associated proteins. In situations where this is not the case, however, T lymphocytes able to infiltrate the tumor tissue have been isolated. These cells have served as the germs for large in vitro cultures and, once mass-produced, have been infused back into the patient. Despite this accomplishment, dramatic improvements have been observed in very few patients.

Directing monoclonal antibodies against molecules present on the surface of tumor cells is an alternative solution—although this strategy, too, has achieved only limited success. Antibodies against the interleukin-2 receptor, which is normally found in cancers caused by the AIDS-related virus HTLV-1, can bring about remission. But in other tumors, prior treatment to reduce the tumor mass—either surgically or with other therapies—is a necessary prerequisite for such success.

Yet another promising line of attack exists. Immunologists have been able to elicit both the humoral and cell-mediated responses using hybrid molecules: artificial structures that combine the features of other immunologically relevant molecules. One interesting hybrid consists of an anti-tumor antibody and a superantigen. Superantigens are proteins of mostly microbial origin that have a unique ability to activate a substantial proportion of T lymphocytes, regardless of their antigen specificity. The antibody part of the compound can bind to antigens on the tumor surface. The superantigen part of the molecule recruits large numbers of T cells to attack the tumor cells (the T cells "think" they are attacking the superantigen). In tests, such antibody-superantigen hybrids have been able to bring about the destruction of tumor cells (see Figure 9.6).

In addition to protecting against disease, antibodies can be converted into highly potent antigens capable of provoking a strong immune response. In the 1960s Jacques Oudin of the Pasteur Institute showed that some antibodies could be recognized by other antibodies as antigens. Oudin called such antigens "idiotypic" and the antibodies that reacted with them "anti-idiotypic." The concept of antibodies and anti-antibodies was extended by the Danish Nobel laureate Niels K. Jerne into a vision of immunologic networks. In such a system, some anti-idiotypic antibodies react with the antigen-binding site of the idiotypic antibody and look like the antigen itself. Although Jerne's work was initially treated with skepticism, it has now been shown that anti-idiotypic antibodies may indeed function like the antigen they mimic. They can therefore foster active and protective immunity against an infectious disease.

Antibodies may even be designed to take over functions of antigens or antigenic molecules. One of the first reports of such an expanded function came from experiments on insulin antibodies. Antibodies that can arise against insulin were used to produce anti-antibodies. When these anti-antibodies were tested for biological activity, it was found that they reacted with antibodies against insulin, thereby blocking attacks on insulin. Most important, they were also found to bind to cellular receptors for insulin, and when given to animals, they lowered blood glucose levels. In other words, some of the anti-antibodies functioned like insulin (see Figure 9.7).

Antibody molecules were later shown to be capable of mimicking the function of several other molecules, including neurotransmitters and regulatory molecules in the immune system. Although these findings have not yielded clinically useful treatments, this situation may change soon. In a remarkable series of studies, it has been possible to produce antibodies with enzymatic, or catalytic, capacity.

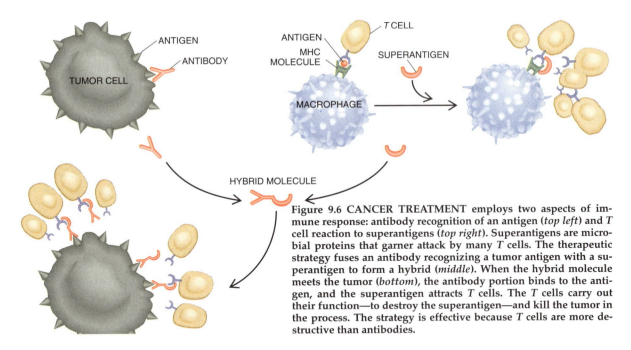

Figure 9.6 CANCER TREATMENT employs two aspects of immune response: antibody recognition of an antigen (*top left*) and *T* cell reaction to superantigens (*top right*). Superantigens are microbial proteins that garner attack by many *T* cells. The therapeutic strategy fuses an antibody recognizing a tumor antigen with a superantigen to form a hybrid (*middle*). When the hybrid molecule meets the tumor (*bottom*), the antibody portion binds to the antigen, and the superantigen attracts *T* cells. The *T* cells carry out their function—to destroy the superantigen—and kill the tumor in the process. The strategy is effective because *T* cells are more destructive than antibodies.

These catalytic antibodies can extend the range of antibody activity, allowing them to do more than bind to a target. The enzymatic activities performed by such antibodies include the cleavage of conventional peptide bonds, as well as entirely new functions, such as the detoxification of highly poisonous molecules. Toward that end, a team led by Donald Landry at Columbia University College of Physicians and Surgeons recently designed a catalytic antibody that can break down cocaine in the bloodstream. Immunologists may soon be able to create proteases with the ability to split selectively an essential envelope protein present on an otherwise lethal virus such as HIV. Because antibodies have a comparatively long half-life in vivo, enzymatically active antibodies could be used to replace a missing enzyme.

Although the predominant approach to designing immunotherapies has been based on the antigen-specific elements of the immune system—antibodies and *T* cells—the picture is rapidly changing. The isolation, cloning, expression and production of a great many pharmacologically active polypeptides and proteins from the more ancient, antigen-nonspecific parts of the immune system have resulted in a novel channel for medical investigations.

During evolution, our immune system developed an intricate set of devices to disarm infections. For instance, small peptides, called cecropins, defensins and magainins, are sometimes found in the skin and mucous membranes of higher animals as well as in insects. These peptides destroy many bacteria by inserting themselves into the bacterial wall and breaking it down.

Investigators have recently determined that slight alterations in the composition of these peptides do not impair their function. Peptides can be made synthetically of amino acids that orient to the right, referred to as D-amino acids, instead of to the left, as they normally do. (L-amino acids, or those that have a leftward orientation, are the biologically active amino acids found in our bodies.) Surprisingly, these D-amino acid peptides have the same effects as their mirror images, are more stable and less easily degraded. This discovery suggests that the D-peptides are not binding to receptors—otherwise, they would not have any activity—but rather to lipids specific to the bacterial wall. Therefore, researchers may be able to produce long-lasting self-based antibiotics that can kill bacteria but not harm the cells of the host.

Other pharmacologically active proteins offer other possibilities for therapies. In particular, a family of proteins called cytokines are of interest.

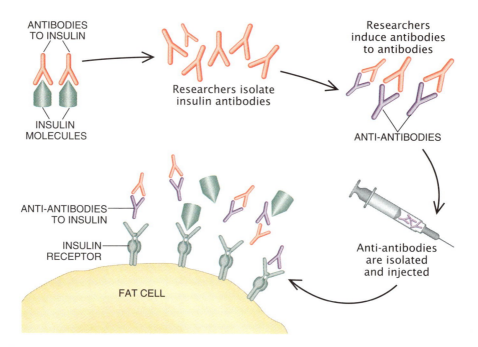

Figure 9.7 ANTIBODIES TO ANTIBODIES can be used to mimic biological substances and to curb immune responses. In some disease states, the immune system creates antibodies to insulin (*red figures at top left*). Such antibodies can be harvested in the laboratory (*center*) and used to provoke the production of anti-antibodies (*purple figures at top right*). When introduced into a patient (*bottom*), anti-antibodies block the antibodies that harm insulin. They also bind to the insulin receptor and cause blood glucose levels to drop.

This family comprises the interleukins, which are produced by white blood cells, and interferons, which stimulate the activity of lymphocytes and scavenger cells that digest foreign particles.

Interferons were the first such chemicals to be molecularly defined. They received their name from the clinical observation that a patient infected with one virus appeared to be protected against a second one because some immunologic feature interfered with the virus's reproduction. There are three major types of interferons: alpha, beta and gamma.

After a series of overenthusiastic claims by researchers, interferons are now finding their place as more conventional drugs to treat some viral diseases—among them chronic hepatitis *B* and C, larynx papillomas and relatively rare tumors, such as hairy-cell leukemias and carcinoids of the gut. Lately some remarkably positive results have emerged from the treatment of multiple sclerosis with beta-interferon, although the reasons for these results are unclear. Gamma-interferon treat-

ment in this disease has the opposite effect of deterioration.

Although it is somewhat painful for a scientist to admit, the underlying effector mechanism used by interferons in individual diseases is for the most part unknown. Therefore, new applications for interferons may stem from trial-and-error studies rather than from precise interventions based on scientific knowledge. Nevertheless, I anticipate that interferons will find an increasing number of applications in the clinic, especially in the field of tumor treatment.

It is beyond the scope of this chapter to enter into a thorough analysis of interleukins: the number of defined interleukins is soon expected to exceed 20. But enough is known about several of these chemicals so that some speculative predictions can be made. The inclusion of some interleukins or their precursors in more conventional types of vaccines against infectious diseases has, in experimental systems, been shown to have profound consequences on the composition and the intensity of the subsequent immune response. In some instances, the simultaneous production in the local tissue of the antigens of the vaccine vector and the interleukin could synergize, inducing an enhanced and focused immune response against the antigens.

The occurrence of interleukins in infectious disease is not an insignificant issue. In two parasitic diseases, namely, schistosomiasis and African sleeping disease, it has been found that induction of two cytokines—tumor necrosis factor-alpha and gamma-interferon, respectively—are essential for parasite colonization. It is thus essential that vaccines that induce immunity not only enhance the production of some cytokines but also avoid the induction of others. Our understanding of these powerful compounds will continue to progress through studies of pure interleukins, transgenic mice that overexpress a single interleukin and so-called knockout mice that do not express an interleukin.

The discovery of new forms of treatments, such as those that include cytokines, shows us that the human immune system has riches as yet unearthed. The complexity of this defensive system promises a wealth of proteins and molecular strategies that can continue to forge medical innovation. And, like miners equipped with brighter headlights and sharper picks, immunologists can select and extract these treasures with increasing ease.

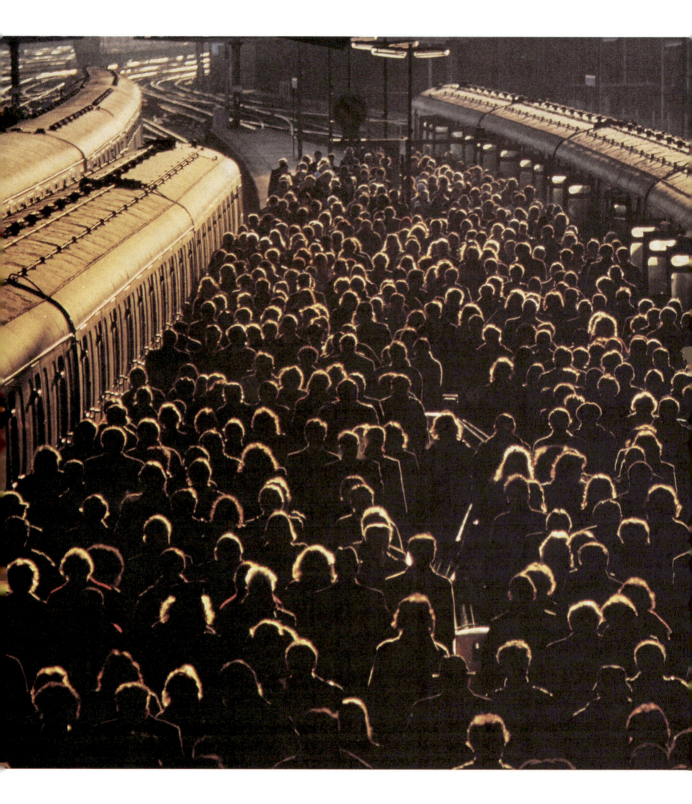

Will We Survive?

As host and pathogen evolve together, will the immune system retain the upper hand?

· · ·

Avrion Mitchison

The human species has existed in something like its present form for about 200,000 years. During that time, the immune system has presumably played a crucial role in our ability to weather exposure to parasites, bacteria, viruses, toxins and other hazards that assert themselves by interacting with our biochemistry. The relationship, one must note, has been an ongoing, mutual one in which all parties have adapted to each other through a variety of means, from open warfare to accommodation and even symbiosis. As the relationship has proceeded, neither we nor our cohabitants have stood still in an evolutionary sense. Such a long run should by itself give us confidence that our species will continue to survive, at least insofar as the microbial world is concerned. Yet such optimism might easily transmute into a tune whistled whilst passing a graveyard.

Changes in some key aspects of humanity's conditions of existence have created the uncertainty. As a result, our immune system has never before

faced more daunting challenges. For perhaps a century—a trivial amount of time from an evolutionary perspective—about 20 percent of us have lived in modern industrial society, an artificial environment of our own construction, notably free of parasites and many pathogens to which our immune system responds. Good news, perhaps. Yet questions arise concerning the effect underemployment might have on our defenses.

The immune system may no longer enjoy the luxury of time. Air travel, major population growth and the emergence of megacities have vastly increased the ease with which people can become exposed to agents of disease (see Figures 10.1 and 10.2). For their part, the microbes have not been resting on their laurels. New ones continually come into being. A virus now exists that attacks the very defenses on which we rely for survival—the human immunodeficiency virus (HIV). The *Legionella* bacterium, the Lyme disease spirochete and the Rift Valley fever virus also exemplify nature's ability to challenge the immune system radically. Even old pathogens invent new tricks (see Figure 10.3). Recently evolved drug-resistant strains of the tuberculosis bacillus have been plaguing industrial urban centers. Will such developments change the comfortable deadlock? Will *Homo sapiens* and the microbes continue to coexist, or will one side win?

Figure 10.1 CHALLENGE to the immune system is presented by the rapid growth of the human population, the crowding together of many individuals in large cities, such as London (*one of the city's commuter rail stations is shown here*), and the existence of high-speed, efficient means of travel. Such factors change our relationship to viruses, bacteria and parasites.

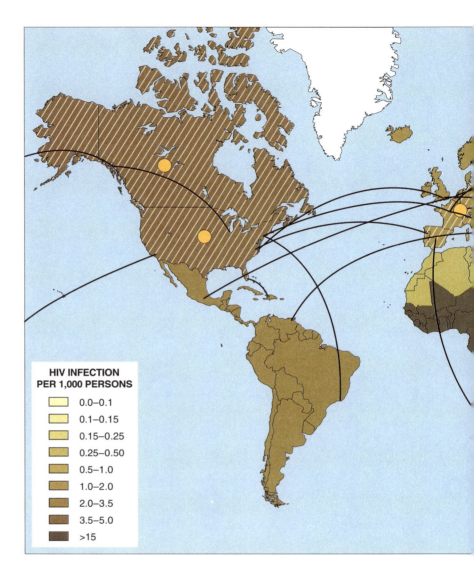

HIV INFECTION
PER 1,000 PERSONS

- 0.0–0.1
- 0.1–0.15
- 0.15–0.25
- 0.25–0.50
- 0.5–1.0
- 1.0–2.0
- 2.0–3.5
- 3.5–5.0
- >15

An important part of the answer to that question can be found in the evolutionary history of the immune system. We need to look back over a few hundred million years to when the earliest vertebrates evolved from their invertebrate ancestors, for at that time the immune system first appeared. The inquiry turns up a significant fact: the immune system has always served the sole purpose of defense against infection. No other external factor shaped it. This observation is demonstrated today by those rare experiments of nature in which infants are born with an immune system that does not function because one critical gene has mutated.

If left untreated, these infants will die from infection. They can survive only in a sterile isolator, known as a bubble. The same natural experiment shows that tasks such as protection against aberrant growth within the host do not affect the immune system's development. Bubble babies and their animal counterparts—mice with a congenital thymus defect, for example—

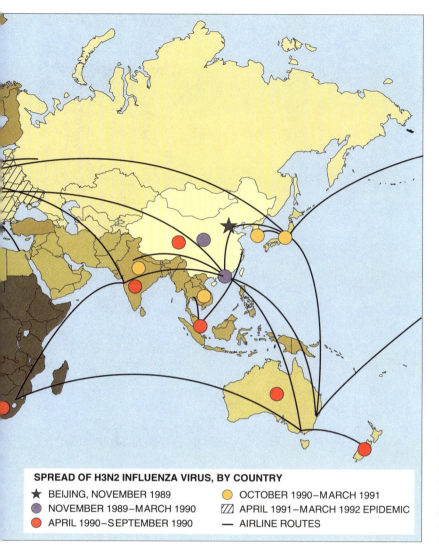

SPREAD OF H3N2 INFLUENZA VIRUS, BY COUNTRY

★ BEIJING, NOVEMBER 1989
⬤ NOVEMBER 1989–MARCH 1990
⬤ APRIL 1990–SEPTEMBER 1990
⬤ OCTOBER 1990–MARCH 1991
▨ APRIL 1991–MARCH 1992 EPIDEMIC
— AIRLINE ROUTES

Figure 10.2 RAPID DIFFUSION OF DISEASE by air travel and other forms of transportation is a fact of contemporary life. Serious, sometimes lethal, infectious diseases such as various strains of influenza, AIDS and new, drug-resistant strains of tuberculosis spread rapidly around the world, often from developing to industrialized countries.

do not have a high incidence of most types of cancer.

These natural experiments eliminate two other suggested functions. Some investigators have proposed that the immune system stimulates the growth of red blood cells. Yet participants in the natural experiment still make normal numbers of erythrocytes. Other workers have proposed that the immune system can prevent some forms of sterility by warding off the effects of paternal leukocytes. Yet mice that have a congenital thymus defect, if kept alive in a semisterile environment, reproduce quite well.

The findings do not necessarily mean that the immune system cannot be made to attack cancer cells or to facilitate reproduction. But one has to be realistic: it will not be easy to persuade the system to perform chores to which it has not grown accustomed in the course of evolution.

In addition to singleness of purpose, consideration of the immune system's history reveals a second major feature: the immune system appears to

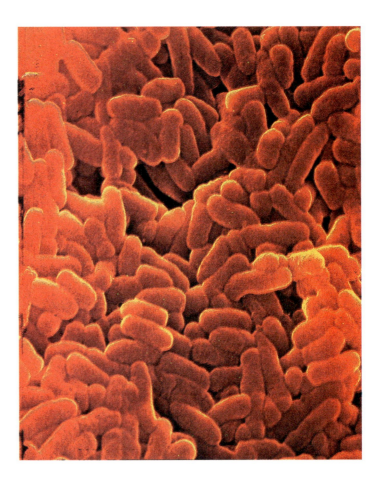

Figure 10.3 NEW TUBERCULOSIS STRAIN is highly virulent and resists drugs. Such altered forms of traditional pathogens as well as such new pathogens as the human immunodeficiency virus (HIV) and *Legionella*, which causes Legionnaires' disease, challenge and even undermine the human immune system.

have evolved through a process of elaboration. It has achieved its protective power by incorporating a variety of defenses that existed in the invertebrates. It did not merely override those mechanisms and replace them with something better.

Among the perfectly serviceable systems that protect invertebrates are wandering phagocytic cells as well as proteins, floating freely in body fluids, that can bind to invading bacteria. These defenses can perform most tasks of the full-fledged immune system, except for mounting heightened responses against organisms that are previous invaders. The ancient defenses have no specific memory—a hallmark of the immune system proper.

Having evolved in the presence of these older, nonadaptive defenses, the immune system incorporates some of their elements for its own purposes. It is not fanciful to trace the modern complement system or antigen-presenting cells back to these ancestral forms. One finds such ancient molecules as complement receptors on modern lymphocytes. Our macrophages sport major histocompatibility complex (MHC) molecules—structures derived from the phagocytic cells of invertebrates.

The immune system seems to have created its ability to recognize antigens and to mount attacks against them by evolving from and incorporating "dumb" defensive proteins such as complement. The nervous system evolved in much the same way. It probably became more intricate to carry out more complex functions. Thus, the oldest part, the brain stem, mediates automatic functions, such as heartbeat and breathing. The cerebellum governs complex motor movements, whereas the cerebrum functions as the seat of consciousness, mediates perception and coordinates the whole.

The resemblance between the two systems extends to structure as well as function. A cytoskeleton consisting of its characteristic array of specialized proteins can be recognized in organisms as primitive as yeast. The cytoskeleton does more than passively support the cell's structure. In our neurons, for example, it serves as the machinery that moves vesicles containing transmitters from the cellular interior to the synapse. In the immune system, antigen-presenting cells, using a similar method, are able to ingest foreign material, break it down and present its essential components to the exterior world.

Unfortunately, we cannot trace most of the evolutionary steps that the immune system took. Virtually all the crucial developments seem to have happened at an early stage of vertebrate evolution, which is poorly represented in the fossil record and from which few species survive. Even the most primitive extant vertebrates seem to rearrange their antigen receptor genes and possess separate T and B cells, as well as MHC molecules. Thus has the immune system sprung up fully armed. It is regrettable that so few of the evolutionary experiments of the transition to vertebrates seem to have survived.

Only for the immunoglobulins can we discern much of an evolutionary story. Presumably, the first system comprised but a single immunoglobulin-producing gene. It quickly re-created itself, establishing a series of duplicates, each making a different immunoglobulin molecule. Then control mechanisms emerged that could direct the production of separated gene segments that were able to recombine. Yet even humans retain in a corner of their immune system something of the primitive arrangement: the genes that control the production of the lambda light-chain immunoglobulin, one form of which consists of only two members.

Molecules of immunoglobulin, the proteins most characteristic of the immune system, combine with antigen to flag its presence to other leukocytes or to initiate destructive chain reactions of complement. Such proteins can be grouped into superfamilies. The fruit fly, *Drosophila*, has been found to employ molecules that resemble those of the immunoglobulin superfamilies. Their role, however, is not immunologic. As cellular adhesion molecules, they guide the growth of neurons in larvae.

Some immunologically significant molecules are even older. Bacteria, for example, have transporter proteins. These proteins are homologous to those that our own cells use to carry peptides to MHC molecules. There the proteins load the peptides into the antigen-presenting groove. The cogent feature of the immune system is that its proteins have diversified and specialized to an extent unprecedented, except in the nervous system. Only a very few of the molecules of the immune system are really new. Natural selection—in Francis Crick's words, the "tinkerer"—needs only a limited number of parts in its erector set.

Recent research on the immune systems of fish and amphibians has identified another interesting survival. These cold-blooded vertebrates have relatively slow-acting immune systems, equipped with poorly diversified antigen receptors. The tadpole of the common frog, for example, makes only about 100 different antibody molecules. On the other hand, frogs have potent defense peptides, called magainins, that punch holes in bacterial cell walls. Molecules that function as magainins do, such as the squalamines of sharks and the cecropins made by insects (and perhaps by many other species) have been found throughout the animal kingdom—even in warm-blooded creatures.

The immune system, then, probably passed much of its early life in a sluggish, relatively inefficient style, playing a fairly minor role in defense. The system came fully into its own only much later on, after the revolution of warm-bloodedness enabled our cells to multiply rapidly.

As the immune system grew in importance and complexity, it underwent a series of internal reorganizations, which involved compromises or trade-offs of one kind or another. The fact that the metabolic resources of an organism are not unlimited makes such economic choices necessary. Investment in effector systems, the cutting edge where killer cells and antibodies wallop bacteria and viruses, must be balanced by investment in regulatory systems necessary for keeping the entire enterprise under control. Thus, in the human immune system there are more regulatory T cells, known as CD4 cells, than any other kind.

One cannot avoid the language of capitalism here, any more than one can in discussing ethology. Immunologists will surely follow in the footsteps of those colleagues who have for quite a while been discussing the investment of deer in antlers or the advantage of balance to hummingbirds in finding fresh flowers. What a perfect microcosm of the market the lymph nodes and spleen offer. In the germinal centers of these organs, mutating B cells furiously compete with one another for the tiny amount of antigen needed for survival. The winners are assured the reward of massive replication. Cells that do not find antigen die.

Where nature fails to provide evidence to support the inquiry into evolution, immunologists have borrowed a tool from economists: computer modeling. Franco Celada of the Hospital for Joint Diseases in New York City and Philip E. Seiden of the IBM Thomas J. Watson Research Center have formulated a cellular automaton for closely modeling the cellular events that take place within the immune system (see Figure 10.4). Sets of simulated T cells, B cells and antigen-presenting cells appropriately endowed with receptors and MHC molecules are (metaphorically) shaken up with antigen and then allowed to undergo a series of interactions. The automaton responds well to antigenic stimulation, mounting recognizable primary and secondary responses.

More interesting results come when it is asked deeper questions—for example, how many MHC types per individual are optimal? The program answers by balancing the advantage of being able to present more and more peptide against the disadvantage of deleting more and more of the T cell repertoire. Recall that in addition to presenting antigen, the MHC molecule identifies tissue as self. So an increase in the number of MHC molecules means an increase in the number of self-antigens. A corresponding number of T cells must therefore be deleted if autoimmunity is to be avoided. Furthermore, loss of MHC types ultimately reduces the flexibility of response to invading organisms.

After a few runs, the model comes up with a number of MHC types between four and eight, which agrees remarkably well with what has been observed. Although not the first mathematical model of the immune system, this is by far the most user-friendly tool available for exploring these evolutionary issues. Its real test will come when it attempts to answer questions to which the solutions are not known.

A related problem is why the antigen-presenting groove in MHC molecules accommodates a sequence of just nine amino acids (see Chapter 3, "How the Immune System Recognizes Invaders," by Charles A. Janeway, Jr.). The hard-nosed biochemist might argue that this size is an accident of the geometry of the MHC molecule. The soft-nosed evolutionary biologist would wonder

whether that explanation alone is sufficient. Instead he or she might argue that the length of the groove may reflect a balance of selective pressure between two opposing needs: on the one hand, to conserve as much of the T cell repertoire as possible and, on the other, to prevent parasites from building proteins invisible to the T cell system. For example, if a groove accommodated only six amino acids, nearly all possible hexapeptides might be present in self-proteins, with the result that nearly all T cells would be deleted. But if a groove accommodated 14 amino acids, parasites could evolve so as to avoid using bindable peptides in their proteins.

One can imagine primitive vertebrates trying out various lengths to find out which one suits best. Testing this possibility lies just beyond the range of present computer models but will surely become possible in the future.

How can one reconcile this tremendous need for economy, and indeed evident economy in so many aspects, with features of the immune system that seem so profligate? Leukocytes, for instance, occur in several repeated sets, each equipped with a more or less complete array of receptors for antigen. We can make a fair guess that the advantage of this repetition lies in allowing specialization. Different immunoglobulins are needed to deal appropriately with different parasites (IgA, say, is the one most effective against worms in the gut), and each immunoglobulin requires its own clone of B cells. Similarly, cytotoxic T cells provide an appropriate defense against viruses such as influenza and intracellular bacteria such as Listeria. And the larger division into T cells and B cells reflects, at least in part, the advantage of giving to the former responsibility for self-tolerance and thereby permitting the latter to indulge in hypermutation. It would never work to combine the two. Imagine the T cell population's getting purged of self-reactive cells in the thymus (which does happen) and then generating new receptors by hypermutation (which happens only to B cells); disastrous autoimmunity would ensue!

We can now begin to derive some answers to our question. I would like to do so by dispelling a possible misconception. So far this account of the evolution of the immune system might suggest that the process had mostly played itself out long ago. In fact, the reverse is true. The human immune system is almost certainly now evolving

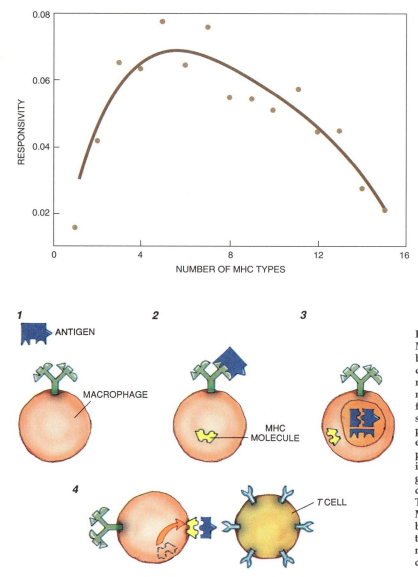

FIGURE 10.4 OPTIMAL NUMBER OF MHC TYPES derives from a balance between the need to respond to a large quantity of invading organisms and the need to avoid autoimmunity. The optimal number of MHC types is between four and eight. The MHC molecule presents antigen to helper *T* cells, and the process begins when a macrophage encounters an antigen (*1*). The macrophage engages the antigen and engulfs it (*2, 3*). When the antigen has been ingested, the cell breaks it down and combines it with an MHC molecule (*4*). The macrophage expresses the antigen-MHC combination on its outer membrane (*lower right*), where it can be detected by a *T* cell, which alerts *B* cells to make antibodies that mobilize either component of the immune system.

more rapidly from generation to generation than ever before. Much of this change affects polymorphic genes, genes that express many different forms of the same MHC or antibody molecule. Our immune system is intensely polymorphic, much more so than any other part of the body. These molecules vary from one individual to another to such an extent that a single combination is hardly ever duplicated. This state of affairs reflects the fact that our parasites breed far more rapidly than we do and can therefore evolve more rapidly.

As with other forms of polymorphism, such as that of wing color in butterflies, this diversity is presumably maintained by selection in favor of heterozygotes. Heterozygotes are individuals that have different copies of each gene, in this case the genes that contribute to the variability of antigen-binding molecules. An individual clearly enjoys an advantage by having, in addition to the four to eight genetic loci mentioned earlier, two different genes at each locus. Such an arrangement maximizes the chances of being able to bind at least one peptide from any one viral or bacterial protein.

Polymorphism in the MHC is indeed more complex and more interesting than simple selection in favor of immune responses to parasites. The reverse also occurs: a vigorous process in all likelihood creates a rich variety of genes whose products suppress the immune response. Such genes are committed to limiting an immune reaction that directly damages the body in the course of responding to a pathogen—they suppress "friendly fire," so to speak (see Chapter 7, "Autoimmune Disease," by Lawrence Steinman).

Nowhere is the balance between the two kinds of control displayed better than in leprosy. The disease afflicts more than one million people in the tropics throughout the world. It disappeared from

Europe only in the past few centuries, for reasons unknown. (Some geographic signs remain. NATO nuclear submarines are based at Lazaretto Point at Holy Loch, so called because of the leprosarium once located there.)

Individuals infected with the leprosy bacterium respond in various ways. Tore Godal of the World Health Organization found that most patients throw off the infection and are left only with traces of reactivity in their immune system (see Figure 10.5). Others acquire a "tuberculoid" infection, in which the body makes a vigorous but only partially effective T cell response. A third group develops a "lepromatous" condition in which the T cell response is suppressed. The skin fills up with

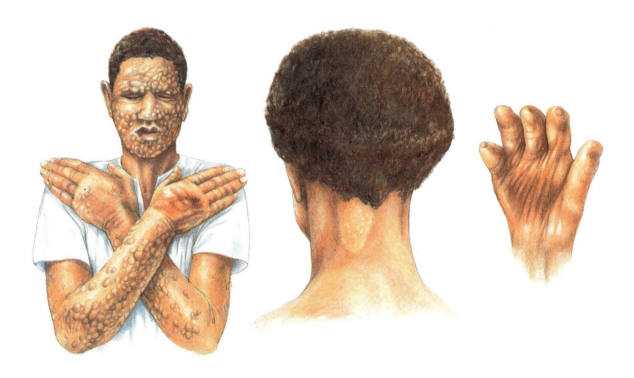

Figure 10.5 LEPROSY, a disease no longer endemic to Europe, shows a range of pathology that is the result of the immune system's ability to shut itself down when the danger exists that a response will damage the host. In the patient at the left, genes are expressed that have led to a lack of effective response. Consequently, the leprosy bacillus multiplies and collects in fluid-filled blebs on the skin. In the patient at the center, an effective immune response has caused no more than a lesion at the hairline. The hand at the right belongs to a patient in whom a vigorous immune response has been mounted but in whom not all the bacteria have been eliminated. In these intermediate cases, the immune response causes tissue damage.

infective bacteria, but life can proceed more or less normally. It is in those cases in which the response has not been so fully suppressed, that immunopathology tends to manifest itself. René de Vries and his colleagues at University Hospital, Leiden, have amply demonstrated that the MHC genes primarily have control of the spectrum of responses.

No doubt these immunosuppressive genes survive in the industrial societies for the most part as relics of chronic infections such as leprosy. In doing so, they provide us (albeit inadvertently) with a measure of protection against the autoimmune and allergic diseases. Donald J. Capra and his associates at the University of Texas Southwestern Medical Center at Dallas conducted a large survey of people suffering from insulin-dependent diabetes who responded to an appeal over the local radio. They found far fewer MHC genes of a specific type (HLA-DQw1.2) within their sample than would have been expected from the frequency in normal control individuals. Presumably, those genes suppress the immune response that destroys the beta cells in a person's pancreas. Similar observations have been made with other HLA genes in other immunologic diseases, such as rheumatoid arthritis and vasculitis.

The protective effect seems hardly large enough to account for the survival of such genes (the diseases are rare and afflict mainly an aged population). They nonetheless excite considerable research interest. At Deutsches Rheuma Forschungszentrum in Berlin, we believe protection is mediated by inhibitory cytokines such as transforming growth factor β. We are searching for treatments that will mimic these genetic effects. In taking this view, we have been much influenced by the pioneering work of Howard L. Weiner of Harvard University on multiple sclerosis, published earlier this year (see Chapter 7, "Autoimmune Disease").

The evolution of immunosuppressive mechanisms is but one example of how hosts and parasites affect one another's development through time; there are many others. Indeed, the more we learn about the molecules of the immune system, the more striking such adaptations appear. Certain viruses, for instance, use molecules of the immune system for gaining access to host cells.

Exploitative in this way as pathogens are, their very cleverness can on occasion be exploited by humankind. John P. Tite and his colleagues at Wellcome Research Laboratories in England have defined a sequence within a bacterial invasin, a protein that facilitates invasion of host tissue. The sequence binds to an integrin, a host–cell surface protein. Tite's group hopes to use this information to build molecules that might block invasin.

Scientists at Immunex Corporation in Seattle have been intrigued by the discovery that certain viruses make cytokine-binding proteins. The proteins increase virulence, presumably by inhibiting the immune response. Immunex workers are building similar proteins in order to combat such autoimmunologic diseases as rheumatoid arthritis (see Figure 10.6).

At the other end of the spectrum, numerous viral DNA sequences have become integrated into the human genome and are never expressed (most of the coat-color varieties prized by fanciers of pet mice result from genes' having been knocked out by just such viral sequences). Or the sequences may get used for purposes that have nothing to do with viral replication. For example, certain viral genes that encode endogenous superantigens have been retained in the genome of the mouse. From that location, they delete the products of other genes called V genes. V genes govern the production of proteins that serve as attachment sites for bacterial superantigens (see Chapter 4, "How the Immune System Recognizes the Body," by Philippa Marrack and John W. Kappler).

One can begin to make sense of this coevolution by considering the principle of the "shared agenda" introduced by Richard Dawkins of the University of Oxford (see boxed figure "Agendas: Shared and Unshared"). The DNA of a dormant endogenous virus has the same needs as the DNA of the host: they share the same agenda almost completely. In contrast, a virus that kills its host after a short latent period has little shared agenda. One ought to add that full dormancy (incorporation into host DNA) is rather unusual, as most viruses do not make reverse transcriptase, the enzyme necessary for incorporation.

The need for transmission of the parasite tends to enforce a common agenda, and almost without exception that is the direction in which evolution has moved. Only new forms of infection, such as viruses that have recently been transmitted from another host species, bring with them their own separate agendas. Seldom if ever does it pay a parasite to kill its host, a fact for which we should be profoundly grateful.

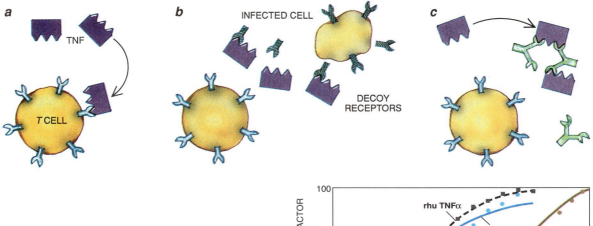

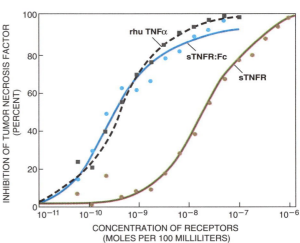

Figure 10.6 THERAPEUTIC STRATEGY for rheumatoid arthritis is suggested by a defensive maneuver the pox virus uses against inflammation. An inflammatory response begins when tumor necrosis factor (TNF) locks onto its receptor (*a*). To block the inflammatory response, viruses lodged in cells that would be destroyed by the reaction cause the production of decoy receptors (*b*), which couple with TNF before the messenger can dock with an immune system cell. Researchers are developing a TNF decoy of two artificial receptors coupled to an antibody fragment. They reason that the Y-shaped assembly will compete effectively for TNF molecules, thereby aborting the autoimmune inflammatory response (*c*). The artificial receptor sTNFR:Fc inhibits response in cultured cells at much lower concentrations than other TNF receptors.

C an we be confident that this tradition of live and let live can persist in the modern world? Opportunities have never been greater for mixing hosts and parasites that have no previous experience of one another. About a billion human beings join the world's population each decade. Many of them crowd into the megacities of the developing countries. High-speed aircraft transportation facilitates the easy movement of millions of people around the globe. The recent past offers illustrations of what can happen when people meet a pathogen from which neither their evolution nor their immune system protects them. One need only recall the English ditty about the malaria-infested west coast of Africa:

The Gulf of Benin, the Gulf of Benin,
Where few come out,
Though many go in.

The mixings of the maritime centuries are a second reason the immune system must be changing more speedily than ever before. Robert C. Gallo of the National Cancer Institute has convincingly argued that HIV probably had its origins in a complex passage of the virus from simians to humans. There is little doubt that the worldwide influenza epidemics have the same kind of origin, starting perhaps when a new variety of virus crosses a species barrier and is then quickly spread around the world by travelers.

Although our cleverness in manipulating the immune system continues to grow in sophistication, our best natural defense against most pathogens, new and old, consists of the immune system's polymorphism. It enables us to counteract the advantage that pathogens enjoy because of their ability to evolve rapidly. So far our storehouse of variability has enabled us to survive.

Agendas: Shared and Unshared

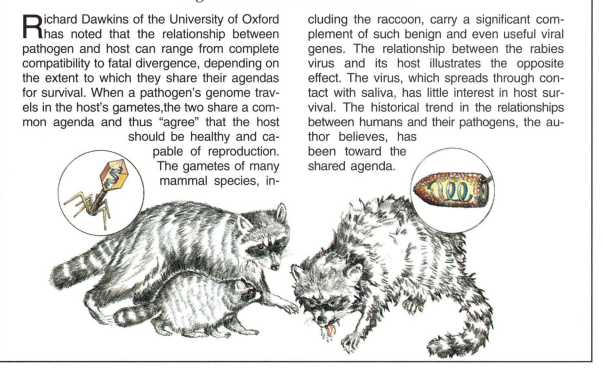

Richard Dawkins of the University of Oxford has noted that the relationship between pathogen and host can range from complete compatibility to fatal divergence, depending on the extent to which they share their agendas for survival. When a pathogen's genome travels in the host's gametes, the two share a common agenda and thus "agree" that the host should be healthy and capable of reproduction. The gametes of many mammal species, including the raccoon, carry a significant complement of such benign and even useful viral genes. The relationship between the rabies virus and its host illustrates the opposite effect. The virus, which spreads through contact with saliva, has little interest in host survival. The historical trend in the relationships between humans and their pathogens, the author believes, has been toward the shared agenda.

Might we count on more radical defenses, such as a further elaboration of structure? Might the control system, for example, arrive at a qualitatively different level of complexity? We cannot count on such a development as a possible further line of defense. All of the existing structures were anticipated in earlier forms of life. And there is no sign that new ones will emerge *ab ovo*.

Rising standards of living and the consequent reduction of the impact of infection on natural selection will be the main forces producing rapid change. We are likely to see in response to the protean challenge of microorganisms variation in the relative frequency of such polymorphic genes as those of the MHC. Later, full-scale gene replacement will occur. Isolation from the complete range of pathogens also enables us to conserve the storehouse of genetic variability that is our chief defense. As long as polymorphisms are unused, they remain available, at the ready, like missiles in their silos.

All these developments should better fit the system for its changing tasks in the modern world.

We can confidently predict that these adaptations will on the whole be beneficial, although just what they will be is unpredictable. We can expect the loss of seemingly deleterious genes to be more conspicuous than the acquisition of beneficial ones.

The possibility even exists that the MHC genes that confer susceptibility to rheumatoid arthritis or multiple sclerosis might gradually disappear. This development would have little to do with any evolutionary effect the diseases might have—after all they afflict older individuals who have had ample opportunity to reproduce. It is more likely to happen because the infections that selected for the maintenance of these genes have been eliminated. From the point of view of an industrialized society, the genes seem harmful, although no doubt they served our infection-riddled ancestors well.

Because we know so little about which MHC genes are needed for which infections, detailed predictions of this kind are difficult. At the start of the *Iliad*, Homer ascribes the plague among the Acheans to arrows shot by the irate Apollo. Would that the god could tell us about the influence of the MHC on his choice of targets!

This overall trend toward a diminishing selection for infection-resistance genes has obvious hazards. As we lower our genetic defenses against the old infections, we will almost certainly increase our susceptibility to new ones. We can comfort ourselves with the knowledge that evolution has moved slowly, maximizing the pros over the cons through many generations, although we need also to remember that human evolution is now moving far faster than ever before.

In comparison with this major trend, other evolutionary forces seem to exert a relatively minor effect. Our growing ability to track the grossly damaging genes mentioned at the beginning of this chapter and to eliminate them through genetic counseling and screening will have an effect that will be more significant for individual families than for the species as a whole. Contraceptive vaccines are in the offing, such as those based on the pregnancy hormone chorionic gonadotropin. G. Pran Talwar and his colleagues at the National Institute of Immunology in Delhi have demonstrated how remarkably effective this form of contraception can be, but only in women who make the right immune response.

Genetic information used appropriately may serve as an even more powerful tool. The better we become at tracing the influence of destructive genetic factors, the better placed we shall be to thwart them. Take rheumatoid arthritis as an example. Studies with twins suggest that genetic factors contribute as much as one third to susceptibility to this disease and that the MHC is the strongest single genetic factor. The situation in diabetes is similar. We can begin to discern a susceptible "type." In the future, we shall be able to draw a much more complete profile of susceptibility, which will no doubt take account of the MHC and other genes as well as such other immunologic parameters as the pattern of cytokine production. All this could be done for healthy individuals, so that they would know in what circumstances to expect their responses to fail or to go too far. They could then take steps to avoid or prevent risk.

Has the immune system, then, reached its apogee after the few hundred million years it has taken to develop? Can it respond in time to the new evolutionary challenges? These perfectly proper questions lack sure answers because we are in an utterly unprecedented situation. Even if we knew how often in the past host species had been wiped out by their parasites, that knowledge would tell us little about ourselves as we stand at present. Yet there are grounds for optimism. Never before have we succeeded in eradicating a disease simply by enhancing the activity of the immune system, as was done with smallpox less than 20 years ago. Never before has science been so sophisticated and so solidly lined up against infections, thanks to the World Health Organization (and more particularly its special research programs) and to such national organizations as the Centers for Disease Control in Atlanta.

But above all, I put my trust in the powers of microevolution, in the capacity of polymorphism to pull new defenses out of its vast storeroom, and in the ability of host and parasite ultimately to adopt a common agenda.

Epilogue

Immunology and Reciprocity

. . .

Barry R. Bloom

Reciprocity, recognized from the time of Confucius as a fundamental value in human relationships, has not usually been regarded as important to the scientific endeavor. Yet few areas of biomedical science have provided greater opportunities for reciprocal interaction between science and the real world than immunology. Basic knowledge of the immune system is clearly essential for informing new efforts to resist infections, to reject tumors and to ameliorate allergies and autoimmune diseases.

In that sense, it is easy to fit immunology into the classical paradigm of the unidirectionality of science, proceeding from the basic to the applied. But it is crucial to appreciate that many of the most practical applications of immunology—diagnostic tests, vaccines and therapeutic interventions—derive from fundamental research undertaken with no obvious practical application in mind. To cite just one example, basic studies of communication between white cells led to identification of the receptor on *T* cells for the AIDS virus.

Many in the scientific community are concerned because society seems to be placing increasing emphasis on solving real-world problems without recognizing that useful applications cannot simply be legislated but depend on basic knowledge not yet acquired. And in modern times, that knowledge has derived from the imaginations of scientists with the freedom to pursue original ideas independent of their perceived immediate utility. If science appears always to lag our needs, it still remains ahead of everything else.

In another sense, however, understanding in immunology has derived from a different paradigm, from a reciprocity with clinical medicine and efforts to master diseases. Studies of children who have rare genetic deficiency diseases that make them highly susceptible to infection, for example, helped researchers to decipher the crucial role of the thymus and antibody-producing cells in immunology.

Through this reciprocity has come the ultimate application of immunology to improving the human condition—vaccines. Economists know it costs much less to prevent disease than to cure it, and vaccines have proved to be one of the most cost-effective interventions to prevent death and disease. In our own country, President Bill Clinton has proposed a comprehensive childhood immunization initiative. The program aims to eliminate an impressive list of diseases by the end of this decade: diphtheria, tetanus, poliomyelitis, measles, rubella, mumps, whooping cough and bacterial meningitis. It would reduce pneumonia and influenza in adults older than 65 years. It will promote the development of immunologic interventions—vaccines in the broadest sense—not only against infectious diseases, such as AIDS, but against allergies, arthritis, multiple sclerosis and cancer.

Beyond the borders of the U.S., more than three million lives have been saved by childhood immunizations. Since 1974 the efforts of UNICEF and the World Health Organization have brought the number of the world's children receiving immunizations by the age of one from 15 to 80 percent. It is shocking that in the U.S. only about half of our children receive their recommended immunizations by the age of two, and in such cities as Houston and Miami that figure is less than 30 percent. At another level for reciprocity, then, we have much to learn from developing countries that protect their children.

In his book *Preparing for the Twenty-First Century*, Paul Kennedy identifies the major issues to be addressed as we head into the next century as equity, population and the environment. In a curious way, immunology may have something to contribute to each. There are enormous disparities in quality of life of people born in different parts of the world. The Third World contains three fourths of the earth's population. There 87 percent of all births and 98 percent of all infant and childhood deaths occur. One in 10 people suffers from a tropical disease; 190 million children are undernourished; and 10 million people die of acute respiratory and diarrheal infections each year.

At the same time, the U.S. acquires many of its raw materials from the Third World. In fact, our trade with developing nations exceeds that with Western Europe and Japan combined and is our most rapid area of growth. In recognition of both the needs and the opportunities, 71 heads of state, an unprecedented number, met at the United Nations in 1990 for the World Summit for Children. They pledged to put the health and education of children at the top of the international agenda. And immunology and vaccines have a special role to play. By the end of the decade paralytic poliomyelitis can be eradicated, neonatal tetanus can be eliminated and measles can be controlled. Although parasites are the largest single source of infection, no vaccine against a human parasite currently exists; clearly, the need is urgent for vaccines against malaria, leishmaniasis and other parasitic diseases.

The argument has often been heard that keeping children alive in the Third World merely increases suffering from poverty and malnutrition. I would point out that in no country have birth rates declined prior to a decline in death rates and that one of the most powerful forces for reduction in fertility is child survival—keeping children alive so that parents know they will be taken care of in old age. In addition to contributing to child survival by preventing infectious diseases, immunology has a more direct impact, through immunization against unique antigens of sperm, eggs or hormones to develop safe and reversible antifertility vaccines.

This winding path leads inevitably to the paramount issue for the next century: the environment. The single most important action that can protect the future of our planet is the reduction of population pressure on the earth's natural resources. This key point about the environment was virtually ignored at the 1992 Earth Summit in Rio de Janeiro.

In reflecting on some of the reciprocities between immunology and the real world, I am ineluctably drawn to the conclusion that biomedical research, if allowed to flourish, has incalculable potential for humane contributions—and to Oscar Wilde's view that "a map of the world without utopia on it is not worth glancing at."

Authors

SIR GUSTAV J. V. NOSSAL ("Life, Death and the Immune System") is director of the Walter and Eliza Hall Institute of Medical Research and professor of medical biology at the University of Melbourne in Australia. He earned his medical degree at the University of Sydney in 1954 and his Ph.D. in immunology from the University of Melbourne in 1960. He has worked at Stanford University, the Pasteur Institute and the World Health Organization; he has held his present post since 1965. Nossal is a foreign associate of the U.S. National Academy of Sciences, a fellow of the British Royal Society and a past president of the International Union of Immunological Societies. His contributions to cellular immunology, particularly the "one cell, one antibody" rule and the discovery of antigen-capturing mechanisms, have been recognized by honors from 12 countries.

IRVING L. WEISSMAN and MAX D. COOPER ("How the Immune System Develops") have been investigating the development of the immune system for more than 25 years. Weissman, a professor of pathology, developmental biology and biology at Stanford University, studies T and B lymphocytes, the central cells of the immune system. His laboratory was the first to isolate stem cells in mice and later colloborated in the isolation of human stem cells. Cooper is a Howard Hughes Medical Institute Investigator at the University of Alabama at Birmingham, where he charts the early development of the immune system in vertebrates and practices clinical immunology. He received a bachelor's degree from the University of Mississippi in 1954 and an M.D. from Tulane University in 1957. Weissman received a bachelor's degree from Montana State University in 1961 and an M.D. from Stanford in 1965.

CHARLES A. JANEWAY, JR. ("How the Immune System Recognizes Invaders") is professor of immunobiology and biology at Yale University and an investigator at the Howard Hughes Medical Institute at Yale. He studied at Harvard University, earning a B.A. in chemistry and, in 1969, an M.D. degree. He trained in medicine at Peter Bent Brigham Hospital in Boston and in immunology at the National Institute for Medical Research in England, the National Institutes of Health and Uppsala University in Sweden. Janeway has been on the Yale faculty since 1977. He has written a textbook on immunobiology with Paul Travers of Birkbeck College, University of London.

PHILIPPA MARRACK and JOHN W. KAPPLER ("How the Immune System Recognizes the Body") have pioneered new techniques for studying tolerance in immune cells. Since 1986 they have both been investigators at the National Jewish Center for Immunology and Respiratory Medicine in Denver, part of the Howard Hughes Medical Institute Research Laboratories. Marrack and Kappler have been married for 19 years.

WILLIAM E. PAUL ("Infectious Diseases and the Immune System") is chief of the laboratory of immunology at the National Institute of Allergy and Infectious Diseases. He graduated with honors from Brooklyn College in 1956 and four years later received his M.D. from the State University of New York Downstate Medical Center. During his distinguished career as a researcher, he has held positions at the National Cancer Institute and the New York University School of Medicine. Paul has served as president of the American Association of Immunologists and of the American Society for Clinical Investigation. He is a recipient of the 3M Life Sciences Award and is a member of the National Academy of Sciences.

WARNER C. GREENE ("AIDS and the Immune System") is director of the Gladstone Institute of Virology and Immunology and professor of medicine, microbiology and immunology at the University of California, San Francisco. He earned his M.D. and Ph.D. in 1977 at the Washington University School of Medicine. He has worked at the National Cancer Institute and at Duke University, where he taught and was an investigator for the Howard Hughes Medical Institute. His research has focused on *T* cell activation and growth and on abnormalities induced by retroviral infection.

LAWRENCE STEINMAN ("Autoimmune Disease") is professor of neurological sciences and pediatrics at the Stanford University School of Medicine. He is also chief scientist for immunology at Neurocrine Biosciences, Inc., in La Jolla, California, which develops therapies based on the interactions of the immune, nervous and endocrine systems. He earned his bachelor's degree in physics from Dartmouth College in 1968 and a degree from Harvard Medical School in 1973. Before joining his current departments, he completed a postdoctoral fellowship in chemical immunology at the Weizmann Institute of Science in Israel and a residency in pediatric neurology at Stanford. He is a recipient of the Senator Jacob Javits Award from the National Institute of Neurological Disorders and Stroke.

LAWRENCE M. LICHTENSTEIN ("Allergy and the Immune System") is professor of medicine and director of the Asthma and Allergy Center at Johns Hopkins University. He earned his M.D. from the University of Chicago in 1960 and completed doctoral studies in microbiology at Johns Hopkins in 1965. He has served at Johns Hopkins in various capacities ever since.

HANS WIGZELL ("The Immune System as a Therapeutic Agent") is professor of immunology at the Karolinska Institute in Stockholm, where he has taught since 1982. He is also director of the Swedish Institute for Infectious Disease Control. After earning an M.D. and a Ph.D. at the Karolinska Institute in 1967, Wigzell became professor of immunology at Uppsala University in 1972. In his spare time, Wigzell has been attempting to grow tropical plants in the cold reaches of Sweden. To date his efforts have been unsuccessful.

AVRION MITCHISON ("Will We Survive?") is scientific director of Deutsches Rheuma Forschungszentrum in Berlin. Mitchison studied zoology as an undergraduate at Magdalen College, Oxford, where his tutor was Sir Peter B. Medawar. Having earned a first-class degree in 1948, he received his doctorate in 1952 and went to Indiana University and Jackson Laboratory in Bar Harbor, Maine, as a Commonwealth Fund Fellow. In the years that followed, he did research, lectured and taught at Edinburgh University, Harvard University, Stanford University and University College, London, where from 1971 until 1991 he was professor of zoology and headed that department. Mitchison has received many honors, including the Paul Ehrlich Prize and the Scientific Medal of the Zoological Society of London. He has published more than 200 research papers.

BARRY R. BLOOM, ("Epilogue") is an investigator at the Howard Hughes Medical Institute of Albert Einstein College of Medicine in the Bronx, New York.

Bibliographies

1. Life, Death and the Immune System

Nossal, G. J. V. 1989. Immunological tolerance: Colloboration between antigen and lymphokines. *Science* 245 (July 14): 147–153.

Silverstein, Arthur M. 1989. *A history of immunology*. Academic Press.

Roitt, I. M. 1991. *Essential immunology*. 7th ed. Blackwell Scientific Publications.

Rose, Noel R., and Ian R. Mackay. 1992. *The autoimmune diseases*. Academic Press.

2. How the Immune System Develops

Von Boehmer, Harald and Pawel Kisielow. 1991. How the immune system learns about self. *Scientific American* 265 (October): 74–81.

Golde, David W. 1991. The stem cell. *Scientific American* 265 (December): 86–93.

Rajewsky, Klaus, and Harald von Boehmer. 1993. Lymphocyte development. *Current Opinion in Immunology* 5 (April): 175–176.

3. How the Immune System Recognizes Invaders

Atkinson, John P., and Timothy Farries. 1987. Separation of self from non-self in the complement system. *Immunology Today* 8 (July/August): 212–215.

Blorkman, Pamela J., et al. 1987. Structure of the human class I histocompatibility antigen, HLA-A2. *Nature* 329 (October 8–14): 506–512.

Litman, Gary W., et al. 1993. Phylogenetic diversification of immunoglobulin genes and the antibody repertoire. *Molecular Biology and Evolution* 10 (January): 60–72.

Weiss, Arthur. 1993. T cell antigen receptor signal transduction: A tale of tails and cytoplasmic protein-tryosine kinases. *Cell* 73 (April 23): 209–212.

4. How the Immune System Recognizes the Body

Billingham, R. E., L. Brent and P. B. Medawar. 1953. Actively acquired tolerance of foreign cells. *Nature* 172 (October 3): 603–606.

Kappler, J. W., N. Roehm and P. Marrack. 1987. T cell tolerance by clonal elimination in the thymus. *Cell* 49 (April 24): 273–280.

Goodnow, C. C., S. Adelstein and A. Basten. 1990. The need for central and peripheral tolerance in the B cell repertoire. *Science* 248 (June 15): 1373–1379.

Schwartz, R. H. 1990. A cell culture model for T lymphocyte clonal anergy. *Science* 248 (June 15): 1349–1356.

Ohashi, P. S., et al. 1991. Ablation of "tolerance" and induction of diabetes by virus infection in viral antigen transgenic mice. *Cell* 645 (April 19): 305–317.

5. Infectious Diseases and the Immune System

Mims, Cedric A. 1987. *The pathogenesis of infectious disease*. Academic Press.

Ada, Gordon L. 1989. Vaccines. In *Fundamental immunology*, ed., William E. Paul. Raven Press.

Doherty, P. C., W. Allan, M. Eichelberger and S. R. Carding. 1992. Roles of αβ and γδ cell subsets in viral immunity. *Annual Review of Immunology* 10:128–151.

Sher, A., and R. L. Coffman. 1992. Regulation of immunity to parasites by *T* cells and *T* cell–derived cytokines. *Annual Review of Immunology* 10:385–409.

Kaufmann, Stefan H. E. 1993. Immunity to intracellular bacteria. *Annual Review of Immunology* 11:129–163.

6. AIDS and the Immune System

Greene, Warner C. 1991. The molecular biology of human immunodeficiency virus type 1 infection. *New England Journal of Medicine* 324 (January 31): 308–317.

Feinberg, Mark B., and Warner C. Greene. 1992. Molecular insights into human immunodeficiency virus type-1 pathogenesis. *Current Opinion in Immunology* 4 (August): 466–474.

Pantaleo, Giuseppe, et al. HIV infection is active and progressive in lymphoid tissue during the clinically latent stage of disease. *Nature* 362 (March 25): 355–358.

Haynes, B. F. 1993. Scientific and social issues of human immunodeficiency virus vaccine development. *Science* 260 (May 28): 1279–1286.

Weiss, Robin A. 1993. How does HIV cause AIDS? *Science* 260 (May 28): 1273–1279.

7. Autoimmune Disease

Oldstone, M. B. 1987. Molecular mimicry and autoimmune disease. *Cell* 50 (September 11): 819–820.

Wraith, David C., Hugh O. McDevitt, Lawrence Steinman and Hans Acha-Orbea. 1989. *T* cell recognition as the target for immune intervention in autoimmune disease. *Cell* 57 (June 2): 709–715.

Springer, Timothy A. 1990. Adhesion receptors of the immune system. *Nature* 346 (August 2): 425–434.

Nepom, Gerald T., and Henry Erlich. 1991. MHC class-II molecules and autoimmunity. *Annual Review of Immunology* 9: 493–525.

Steinman, Lawrence. 1991. The development of rational strategies for selective immunotherapy against autoimmune demyelinating disease. *Advances in Immunology* 49: 357–379.

8. Allergy and the Immune System

Kay, A. Barry, K. Frank Austen and Lawrence M. Lichtenstein, eds. 1984. *Asthma: Physiology, immunopharmacology, and treatment*. Academic Press.

Middleton, E., Jr., C. E. Reed, E. F. Ellis, N. F. Adkinson and J. W. Yunginger, eds. 1988. *Allergy: Principles and practice*. C. V. Mosby.

Valentine, Martin D., et al. 1990. The value of immunotherapy with venom in children with allergy to insect stings. *New England Journal of Medicine* 323 (December 6): 1601–1603.

Bochner, Bruce S., and Lawrence M. Lichtenstein. 1991. Anaphylaxis. *New England Journal of Medicine* 324 (June 20): 1785–1790.

Charlesworth, E. N., W. A. Massey, A. Kagey-Sobotka, P. S. Norman and L. M. Lichtenstein. 1992. Effect of H_1 receptor blockade on the early and late response to cutaneous allergen challenge. *Journal of Pharmacology and Experimental Therapeutics* 262 (September): 964–970.

Togias, A. G., and L. M. Lichtenstein. 1992. The pathophysiology of allergic rhinitis and its implications for management. In *The mast cell in health and disease*, eds., M. A. Kaliner and D. D. Metcalfe. Marcel Dekker.

9. The Immune System as a Therapeutic Agent

Klein, Jan. 1990. *Immunology*. Blackwell Scientific Publications.

Osterhaus, A. D., and F. G. Uytedehaag. 1990. *Idiotype networks in biology and medicine: Proceedings of the international conference on idiotype networks in biology and medicine*. Elsevier Science Publications.

Ginsberg, Harold S., et al., eds. 1993. *Vaccines 93: Modern approaches to new vaccines including prevention of AIDS*. Cold Spring Harbor Laboratory Press.

10. Will We Survive?

Mitchison, N. A. 1990. The evolution of acquired immunity to parasites. *Parasitology* 100, supplement: S27–S34.

———1992. Specialization, tolerance, memory, competition, latency, and strife among *T* cells. *Annual Review of Immunology* 10:1–12.

———1993. A walk round the edges of self tolerance. *Annals of Rheumatic Diseases* 52, supplement 1 (March): S3–S5.

———1993. *T*-cell activation states: The next breakthrough in signaling? *Immunologist* 1 (May/June): 78–80.

Sources of the Photographs

J. Bertrand/Leo de Wys, Inc.: Figure 1.1
Bettmann Archive: Figure 1.2
Peter M. Colman and William R. Tulip, CSIRO: Figure 1.3
Tom Mandel and Rosie van Driel, Walter and Eliza Hall Institute of Medical Research: Figure 1.5 (*top*)

Robert Becker/Custom Medical Stock: Figure 2.1

Don Fawcett/Science Source, Photo Researchers, Inc.: Figure 3.1
Paul Travers, Birkbeck College, University of London: Figure 3.4

CNRI/Science Photo Library, Custom Medical Stock: Figure 4.1
R. D. Owen, H. P. Davis and R. F. Morgan, *Journal of Heredity* 37 (October 1946): Figure 4.2

Peter Charlesworth/J. B. Pictures: Figure 5.1

NIBSC/SPL, Photo Researchers, Inc.: Figure 6.1
George Washington University: Figure 6.2 (*bottom*)
Anthony S. Fauci, National Institute of Allergy and Infectious Diseases: Figure 6.3

Rahul Mehta and Dieter Enzmann, Stanford University School of Medicine: Figure 7.1 (*MRI scans*)
Moses Rodriguez, Mayo Foundation: Figure 7.2
Stanford Visual Arts Service: Figure 7.4

Dan Wagner: Figure 8.1
Ann M. Dvorak, Harvard Medical School: Figure 8.2
St. Bartholomew's Hospital, London/SPL, Photo Researchers, Inc.: Figure 8.3
Jeremy Burgess/SPL, Photo Researchers, Inc.: Figure 8.4

Max Aguilera-Hellweg; courtesy of University of California, San Francisco, Medical Center Liver Transplant Services: Figure 9.1
UPI/Bettmann Newsphotos: Figure 9.2
James Holmes, Cell Tech Ltd./SPL, Photo Researchers, Inc.: Figure 9.3

David Harding/Tony Stone Images: Figure 10.1
CNRI/SPL, Photo Researchers, Inc.: Figure 10.3

INDEX

Page numbers in *italics* indicate illustrations.